Data-Driven Reproductive Health

Abhishek Sengupta • Priyanka Narad
Gaurav Majumdar • Deepak Modi
Editors

Data-Driven Reproductive Health

Role of Bioinformatics and Machine Learning Methods

Springer

Editors
Abhishek Sengupta
Amity Institute of Biotechnology
Amity University Uttar Pradesh
Noida, India

Priyanka Narad
Division of Development Research
Indian Council of Medical Research
New Delhi, Delhi, India

Gaurav Majumdar
Center of IVF and Human Reproduction
Sir Ganga Ram Hospital
New Delhi, India

Deepak Modi
Department of Molecular and
Cellular Biology
National Institute for Research in
Reproductive and Child Health
Mumbai, Maharashtra, India

ISBN 978-981-97-7450-0 ISBN 978-981-97-7451-7 (eBook)
https://doi.org/10.1007/978-981-97-7451-7

This Springer imprint is published by the registered company Springer Nature Singapore Pte Ltd.
The registered company address is: 152 Beach Road, #21-01/04 Gateway East, Singapore 189721, Singapore

Preface

In the past decade, data has taken the forefront. Technology advancements have aided in our understanding of complex biological processes such as reproductive health, where the combination of bioinformatics and machine learning has made substantial progress. Reproductive health is a complex biological process, and data-driven approaches would aid in several aspects of better comprehension. The combination of bioinformatics and machine learning methods has significantly contributed to the progress in this field. By leveraging large datasets and advanced analytical tools, researchers and healthcare professionals can gain deeper insights into the complexities of reproductive health. Utilizing bioinformatics, researchers can effectively analyze genomics, transcriptomics, proteomics, and metabolomics data to gain a comprehensive understanding of the molecular mechanisms underlying reproductive health. By uncovering patterns and correlations within the immense amounts of multi-omics biological data, bioinformatics tools enable the identification of potential genetic markers, gene expression profiles, and metabolic pathways associated with fertility, pregnancy complications, and reproductive disorders. An understanding of the process of data mining and information on different repositories and types of reproductive health data would provide a modern outlook for the analysis of this complex data. Most of the previous resources examine the broad theoretical understanding of reproductive medicine, with a specific emphasis on the biological and public health aspects related to reproductive health. Several sources discuss the advantages of using machine learning techniques in the healthcare field, without specifically addressing reproductive health.

The objective of this book is to provide comprehensive insights into the use of bioinformatics and machine learning methodologies in the analysis of reproductive data for efficient biomarker development, drug discovery, and prediction of diseases and infections. This book provides a thorough dive into the end-to-end process of data-driven reproductive health, highlighting the role of bioinformatics and systems biology. It delves into various crucial aspects related to analyzing reproductive health data, from understanding data sources and preprocessing techniques to exploring advanced methodologies such as multi-omics approaches. This book has been written considering the demand for researchers and students looking to study the methods of data mining and analysis in the field of reproductive health. It consists of practical case studies to illustrate real-world applications. Additionally, this book looks ahead to emerging trends and future directions in the field, making it a valuable resource for researchers, practitioners, and students interested in data-driven approaches in reproductive health analysis. It includes many figures and illustrations for a better and clearer understanding. While the technical content of this book may be more suited for professionals, individuals with a general interest in reproductive health and an inclination toward understanding how data and technology influence healthcare could find this book insightful. Universities and educational institutions offering courses in fields like bioinformatics, data science, public health, and reproductive biology could use this book as a supplementary resource for their curricula.

We are confident that this book will be a valuable resource for readers seeking to understand the broad aspects of data-driven approaches in reproductive health. We look forward to the valuable suggestions and feedback from readers regarding the content of this book.

Noida, Uttar Pradesh, India	Abhishek Sengupta
New Delhi, India	Priyanka Narad
New Delhi, India	Gaurav Majumdar
Mumbai, India	Deepak Modi

Contents

About the Editors

Abhishek Sengupta is an Assistant Professor at the Centre of Computational Biology and Bioinformatics, Amity Institute of Biotechnology, Amity University, Uttar Pradesh, Noida. He received his M.Sc. from Nottingham Trent University, UK, and Ph.D. from Amity University, India. He has been actively involved in teaching and research for 15 years in the fields of genome-scale metabolic reconstructions, constraint-based modeling, network biology, systems biology, metabolomics, and flux balance analysis. He has developed a knowledge-based metabolic model of the human energy pool network for predicting the energy availability status of an individual termed HEPNet, accepted and published by the EBI BioModels database. He also contributed to multiple software and databases like TFIS (Transcription Factor Information System), ARTPre (Assisted Reproduction Prediction), PluriMetNet, FertilitY Predictor, and VIRdb (Vitiligo Information Resource database). He is successfully heading the SBDA Research Lab and has published numerous research papers and book chapters in reputed journals like PLoS One, PeerJ, Springer, Elsevier, Frontiers, and Nature Scientific Reports. He is also heading a DBT, Government of India, funded project titled "A Hybrid Bayesian Approach to Address Socio-economic Challenges in Assisted Reproductive Techniques Across the Indian Sub-population Through a Web-Based Implementation." He has also been awarded an international travel grant as a young scientist by DST-SERB, Government of India, to attend a weeklong (July 3–8, 2016) training course on "In Silico Systems Biology" organized by Wellcome Trust, UK, at EMBL-EBI, Wellcome Genome Campus, Hinxton, Cambridge, United Kingdom. He led the technology transfer and licensing of an ML-based software "FertilitY Predictor" to APS Life Tech, Pune, for which copyright was also granted. He has been awarded copyright for the software "ARTPRE: An Online Tool to Predict the Success Rates of Assisted Reproductive Procedures in Indian Subcontinent."

Priyanka Narad is a Scientist at the Division of Development Research within at the Indian Council of Medical Research (ICMR), headquarters in New Delhi. Priyanka Narad holds a Ph.D. in Biotechnology with a specialisation in Bioinformatics and Network Biology. Over the past 13 years, she has also held the position of Assistant Professor at the Center for Computational Biology and Bioinformatics at Amity Institution of Biotechnology, Amity University. Her expertise lies in the fields of stem cell bioinformatics and machine learning. Her professional interests encompass a broad spectrum including machine learning, multi-omics data integration, clinical data analysis, predictive modeling, transcriptomics data analysis, molecular modeling, docking, and MD simulation studies. She has published numerous research articles in well-reputed journals including Nature Scientific Reports, PeerJ, F1000Research, etc. In 2020, she secured a DBT-funded project titled "A Hybrid Bayesian Approach to Address Socio-economic Challenges in Assisted Reproductive Techniques Across the Indian Sub-population through a Web-Based Implementation." She has successfully deployed and supervised various software and databases such as TFIS, ARTPRE, VIRdb, PluriMetNet, and FertilitY Predictor. Moreover, she holds a license for the technology transfer and licensing of FertilitY Predictor software to APS Life Tech, Pune. Her contributions extend to copyrights for two software programs, namely FertilitY Predictor and ARTPRE, both developed under her guidance and supervision during her stay at Amity University, Noida. Recognized for her academic pursuits, she was granted the DST-SERB Young Scientists Travel Award to attend the "Advanced Course on In Silico Systems Biology" held at WellCome Trust Genome Campus, EMBL-EBI, UK.

Gaurav Majumdar is a Chief Embryologist at the Centre of IVF, Sir Ganga Ram Hospital, New Delhi. He stands as one of the pioneering fully trained and certified embryologists in India, having earned his master's degree in clinical embryology from the National University of Singapore in 2001. Subsequently, he received a Ph.D. for his groundbreaking research in Pre-Implantation Genetic Screening for human embryos in 2018. With over two decades of experience in the IVF laboratory, he has played a pivotal role in elevating the standards of the IVF laboratory at the Centre of IVF, SGRH, resulting in outstanding pregnancy and live birth rates. His expertise extends to optimizing embryo culture protocols and ensuring the production of high-quality embryos that contribute to the center's remarkable success rates, with approximately 60% pregnancy rates from predominantly single embryo transfers. He has also developed a highly efficient embryo freezing program, boasting survival rates exceeding 95%. His meticulous approach includes conducting thorough reviews of embryology details from previous failed cycles, providing valuable insights and tailored treatment options, especially for complex and challenging IVF cases. Beyond his contributions to laboratory excellence, he places significant emphasis on patient care, offering compassionate counseling to support patients through the emotional journey of IVF. He is actively involved in teaching and knowledge dissemination, sharing his expertise with fellow embryologists, and contributing to the continuous advancement of the field. His multifaceted contributions encompass scientific innovation, patient-centric care, and educational mentorship. He was awarded the Economic Times' Fertility Award for Best Embryologist of the Year in India in 2019. His achievements, dedication, and expertise make him a respected leader and key figure in the realm of embryology and reproductive medicine.

Deepak Modi is a renowned Scientist whose contributions in the field of reproductive biology and genetics have earned him accolades and recognition globally. Currently associated with the Department of Clinical Research at the National Institute for Research in Reproductive Health, Indian Council of Medical Research, his academic journey began with a Ph.D. in applied biology from the University of Mumbai in 2003, following an M.Sc. in zoology from the University of Bombay in 1995. His extensive academic qualifications laid the foundation for his exceptional research career. His achievements include the prestigious PM Bhargava Oration Award from the Academy of Clinical Embryologists, India, in 2017, the GP Talwar Middle Career Scientist Award from the Indian Society for the Study of Reproduction and Fertility in 2017, and the ICMR-Tilak Venkoba Rao Award for Reproductive Physiology in 2010, among others. With a specialization in reproductive biology and genetics, his research focuses on understanding the mechanisms involved in embryo implantation, identifying factors leading to implantation failure, pregnancy losses, and preterm births, and studying the genetics of male and female infertility and disorders of sex development. His scholarly impact is evidenced by a substantial publication record, including 85 publications and 3 book chapters, covering a wide array of topics in reproductive biology and genetics. His research has made significant contributions to the scientific community, with selected publications in prestigious journals such as The Journal of Maternal-Fetal and Neonatal Medicine, European Journal of Obstetrics & Gynecology and Reproductive Biology, Frontiers in Cell and Developmental Biology, and many more. He has been actively involved in several research projects such as the Immunomodulatory Roles of Homeobox A10 in the Endometrium During Embryo Implantation (DBT-funded project, 2021–2024), the Development of a Microfluidic-Based Tool for Assessing Placental Functions in Pregnancy Disorders (Intramural project, 2023–2027), HOXA10 in the Pathogenesis of Endometriosis (Intramural project, 2023–2025), Epithelial to Mesenchymal Transition in the Process of Embryo Implantation (Intramural project, 2023–2026), and Placenta of Women with Coronavirus Disease 2019 (COVID-19) (Intramural project, 2023–2025). In addition to his research prowess, he actively participates in scientific conferences, seminars, and workshops, where he serves as an invited speaker, panelist, and session chair. His engagements include conferences organized by esteemed institutions such as ISAR, ACE, and the National Academy of Medical Sciences, reflecting his standing as a respected authority in his field.

1 Introduction to Data Mining in Reproductive Health

Shubham Shekhar Mohanty

Abstract

Reproductive health refers to a healthy male or female reproductive system both defined by physical and mental well-being. In the past decade, research on reproductive health has been at the forefront of healthcare research due to awareness and a plethora of studies generated on the same. This chapter serves as an introduction to the process of data mining in reproductive health covering the basic methodology and applications of data mining in reproductive health. Further, the implementation of electronic health records and disease surveillance is discussed as an aid in data analytics using advanced machine learning methods. The chapter further addresses the challenges and ethical considerations associated with data quality, accessibility, and privacy in reproductive health and emphasizes the approaches for handling such challenges. These technologies can transform reproductive health research by enabling better analysis of medical data, personalized medicine, and early detection of diseases. The implications for the future of reproductive healthcare and data mining are vast, promising advancements in personalized medicine and improved patient outcomes.

Keywords

Reproductive health · Data mining · Machine learning · Electronic health records
Predictive analytics · Personalized medicine

S. S. Mohanty (✉)
Department of Biotechnology, Jaypee Institute of Information Technology, Noida, UP, India

A. Sengupta et al. (eds.), *Data-Driven Reproductive Health*,
https://doi.org/10.1007/978-981-97-7451-7_1

1.1 Introduction

Reproductive health refers to a condition in which every aspect of one's physical, mental, and social health is optimal concerning the reproductive system and all of its operations. Both men and women need to maintain good reproductive health, as it involves the overall health of their reproductive systems and their ability to have a satisfying and safe sex life (WHO 2021).

For healthcare professionals to make better judgments regarding a patient's care, data is essential. Healthcare professionals are better able to deliver a comprehensive treatment plan when they have access to a full picture of a patient's medical history. Data collection is essential for improving patient experiences, as it helps providers identify trends and patterns in patient care, leading to better decision-making and improved outcomes (PrognoCIS EHR 2024).

Data mining has become increasingly important in the healthcare industry, as the amount of data produced has surpassed the ability of traditional methods to process and analyze it. By 2025, the healthcare industry is expected to be responsible for producing about 36% of all global data. This massive amount of data can be processed and analyzed using advanced technologies, such as machine learning algorithms, to gain valuable insights and improve patient care.

Reproductive health faces challenges in effectively utilizing large medical datasets, particularly those involving complex relationships between parents and children (such as genetic information, intergenerational health patterns, and familial medical histories). Traditional statistical methods may not always be sufficient for exploring such intricate data. However, the potential of data mining, including machine learning, has been demonstrated in various studies. For instance, previous research has discussed the value of real-world data mining in clinical practice and highlighted the challenges and opportunities for data science in women's health. The importance of this chapter is underscored by its focus on elucidating the barriers within reproductive health research and delving into the capacity of data mining, specifically machine learning, to surmount these impediments.

This chapter seeks to comprehensively explore the pivotal role of data mining in addressing challenges within the realm of reproductive health research. The scope of this chapter encompasses an in-depth examination of the fundamental concepts of data mining, emphasizing its application in healthcare and, more specifically, in the intricate domain of reproductive health. It aims to elucidate how data mining techniques, including classification, clustering, association rules, and prediction, can be effectively employed to analyze large datasets and derive meaningful insights. By exploring the basics of data mining and its relevance in reproductive health, the chapter lays the foundation for understanding the potential impact of advanced technologies such as machine learning in overcoming the limitations of traditional research methods. Furthermore, the chapter delves into real-world applications of data mining in reproductive health, providing a glimpse into how electronic health records, predictive analytics, and disease surveillance can be leveraged to enhance patient care and inform public health policies. As the review unfolds, it also addresses the challenges and ethical considerations associated with data quality, accessibility, and privacy in reproductive health, emphasizing the need for a nuanced approach. Ultimately, this chapter aims to set the stage for subsequent discussions on case studies, success stories, and future directions, offering readers a comprehensive overview of the evolving landscape of data mining in the context of reproductive health.

1.2 Basics of Data Mining

Data mining is the act of examining huge amounts of data to find patterns, trends, and relationships that can be used to solve business problems and make educated decisions (Han and Pei 2012).

It involves the use of mathematical analysis and advanced algorithms to extract useful information from raw data (Minewiskan 2023). Data mining is a multifaceted process that includes steps such as precise selection, skilled preprocessing, transforming treatments, and insightful interpretation (Fig. 1.1).

Key concepts in data mining include patterns—These are recurring patterns in the data that can help identify relationships between variables or predict future trends (Minewiskan 2023). Models are containers that identify the columns used for input, the attribute being predicted, and the parameters that tell the algorithm how to process the data. Models are frequently taught by applying a specific mathematical method to the data, and the patterns discovered during the training process are determined by the training data used, the algorithm used, and how the algorithm is designed (Minewiskan 2023). Data mining relies on big data, which refers to large, unstructured datasets that are often too large for traditional data exploration methods. Big data and advanced computing processes, such as machine learning, are essential for data mining (Twin 2003) and Knowledge Discovery in Databases (KDD)—Data mining is sometimes referred to as KDD, a data science methodology for gathering, processing, and analyzing data. The KDD process is a step-in data mining, where data is collected, preprocessed, and analyzed to identify patterns and relationships.

To evaluate enormous amounts of data and uncover significant patterns, data mining techniques are rapidly being employed in healthcare and reproductive health research. These strategies can help predict future trends and make sound decisions. Classification, clustering, association rules, and prediction are some typical data

Fig. 1.1 Various factors involved in data mining

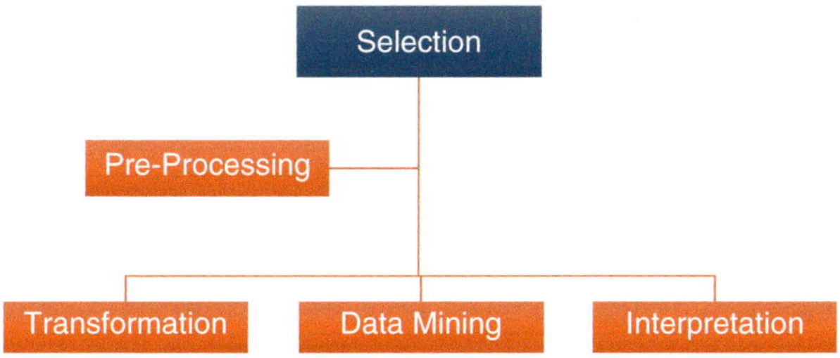

Table 1.1 Data mining techniques in reproductive health research

Technique	Description	Application
Classification	Predicts the likelihood of a specific class membership based on attributes	Predicting risk of reproductive health conditions (e.g., gestational diabetes, preeclampsia)
Clustering	Groups instances based on similarity	Identifying patterns in health patterns among different groups of patients
Association rules	Finds relationships between different attributes or classes	Analyzing patterns of care and relationships between different reproductive health conditions
Prediction	Estimates the value of a target attribute based on other attributes	Predicting fertility levels, onset of reproductive health issues, and effectiveness of treatments

mining techniques used in healthcare (refer to Table 1.1). Classification is used to predict the likelihood of a particular class membership for an instance based on its attributes. In healthcare, classification can be used to predict the risk of a patient developing a certain disease or to categorize patients based on their health status. Clustering is an unsupervised learning technique that groups instances based on their similarity. In healthcare, clustering can be used to identify groups of patients with similar health patterns or to analyze the relationships between different healthcare services. Association rules are used to find the relationships between different attributes or classes in a dataset. In healthcare, association rules can be used to identify patterns of care or to analyze the relationships between different health conditions. Prediction techniques are used to estimate the value of a target attribute based on the values of other attributes. In healthcare, prediction can be used to predict the onset of a disease or to estimate the effectiveness of a treatment (Birjandi and Khasteh 2021).

Some specific applications of data mining in reproductive health research include:

- Utilizing electronic health records (EHR) and insurance claims data to analyze patient health patterns and predict the risk of certain health outcomes (Santos-Pereira et al. 2022).
- Analyzing health datasets gathered from parent-child pairs to explore the causality of reproductive health conditions (Dong et al. 2022).
- Using machine learning techniques to analyze complex reproductive health data and provide valuable suggestions on the feasibility and performance of studies (Dong et al. 2022).

1.3 Applications in Reproductive Health

In the field of reproductive health, electronic health records (EHRs) play a significant role in improving patient care and outcomes. Some applications of EHRs and other data mining techniques in reproductive health include the following.

1.3.1 Electronic Health Records (EHRs)

EHRs are used to store and share patients' pregnancy and abortion care information, allowing healthcare providers to share this data with one another, patients, and third-party applications. This interoperability has become sophisticated enough that documentation and laboratory results can be shared in many circumstances, improving patient care and outcomes (Khanna et al. 2022). EHRs can be used to collect additional information that may be missing or difficult to locate in traditional health records, such as pregnancy outcomes and complications (Bower et al. 2017). This data can be mined to identify trends and patterns, which can help improve patient care and inform public health policies.

1.3.2 Predictive Analytics for Pregnancy and Fertility

Predictive analytics can be used to develop models that help identify factors affecting fertility and improve success rates in assisted reproductive technologies. Data mining techniques can be applied to identify risk factors for pregnancy complications, such as gestational diabetes, preeclampsia, and birth defects. This information can help healthcare providers intervene early and improve patient outcomes.

1.3.3 Disease Surveillance and Epidemiology

EHRs and personal health records (PHRs) can be used to monitor reproductive health trends, such as fertility rates, pregnancy outcomes, and complications (Bower et al. 2017). This data can be analyzed to identify patterns and trends, which can inform public health policies and interventions. Data mining techniques can be used to identify risk factors for various reproductive health issues, such as maternal health complications, preterm labor, and birth defects. This information can help healthcare providers target interventions and improve patient care.

1.4 Methodology

The effective application of data mining in reproductive health research necessitates a well-defined methodology to extract meaningful insights from vast and complex datasets. The process typically involves several key steps. Initially, there is a comprehensive data collection phase, where diverse datasets related to reproductive health, including electronic health records (EHRs), insurance claims, and other pertinent sources, are gathered. Subsequently, data preprocessing is undertaken to address issues such as missing values, outliers, and data normalization, ensuring the data is suitable for analysis. Once the data is prepared, researchers employ various data mining techniques such as classification, clustering, association rules, and prediction to uncover patterns, relationships, and trends within the reproductive health

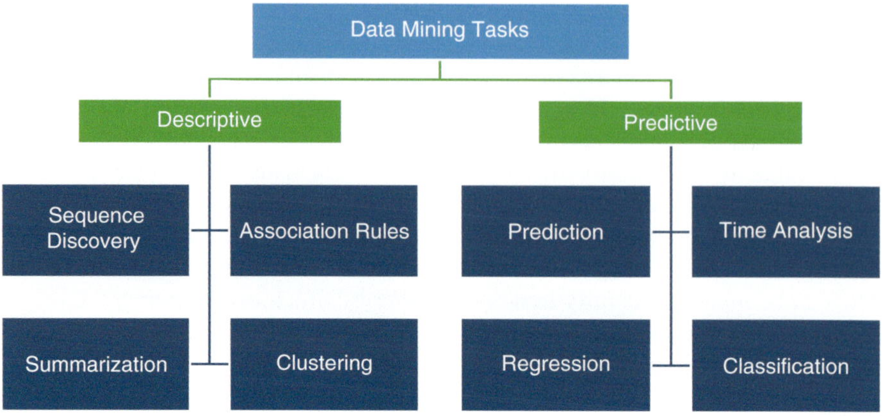

Fig. 1.2 Types of data mining techniques

data (Fig. 1.2). Classification algorithms aid in predicting the likelihood of specific health conditions, while clustering techniques help identify groups of patients with similar health patterns. Association rules reveal relationships between different attributes, offering insights into care patterns and health conditions. Prediction techniques estimate the value of target attributes, enabling the forecasting of fertility levels or the onset of reproductive health issues.

In the field of data mining, there are two main types of techniques that stand out: descriptive and predictive methods. Descriptive techniques involve a range of analytical tools, like sequence discovery, that identify patterns in sequential data like customer behavior or financial transactions. Association rules, crucial for market basket analysis, discover connections between different items in a dataset. Summarization methods effectively condense large amounts of data into brief and manageable summaries, aiding in the comprehension of the information. Cluster analysis, another aspect of descriptive data mining, coordinates the categorization of similar objects according to common characteristics.

On the other hand, predictive data mining methods use past data to predict future occurrences. Forecasting, an essential forecasting method, uses past data to predict future events. Classification is the methodical sorting of data into specific classes based on established criteria. Regression, like other prediction methods, aims to represent the complex connections between a target variable and one or multiple predictors. The examination of time, an important aspect, involves the study of temporal data to identify trends and patterns that develop over time. These varied data mining techniques play a significant role in studying complex datasets, promoting well-informed decision-making and enhancing knowledge across various fields. A crucial aspect of the methodology is the iterative nature of data mining, where initial results may lead to refinement of techniques or revisiting the preprocessing phase. Additionally, the ethical considerations surrounding patient data privacy and the responsible handling of sensitive information are integral components of the methodology. This comprehensive approach ensures that data mining in reproductive health is not only technically sound but also ethically robust, contributing to advancements in healthcare practices and patient outcomes.

1.5 Challenges and Ethical Considerations

The issues related to data quality and accessibility in reproductive health, as well as privacy and ethical concerns, are significant in the context of increasing data sharing and mining applications. Data accessibility and quality in reproductive health are influenced by the increasing desire of for-profit companies to obtain extensive healthcare databases, leading to apprehensions regarding patient privacy and the ethical consequences of disclosing patient data to entities that might misuse it (Chiruvella and Guddati 2021). Additionally, the inadequacy of women's mHealth applications in adhering to fundamental data privacy, sharing, and security norms is a significant worry, especially concerning sensitive reproductive health data (Alfawzan et al. 2022; Chiruvella and Guddati 2021).

Privacy and Ethical Concerns—Privacy issues associated with reproductive health data have been emphasized, particularly in the context of the vast data ecosystem collecting and monetizing all aspects of reproductive health, which is in direct odds with personal secrecy and privacy protection. Furthermore, the ethical and legal implications of sharing patient data with for-profit companies, as well as the lack of basic data privacy and security practices in women's mHealth apps, have raised significant ethical concern (Alfawzan et al. 2022; Chiruvella and Guddati 2021). The intersection of data privacy, ethical concerns, and data accessibility in reproductive health necessitates a comprehensive and nuanced approach to address these complex challenges.

1.6 Case Studies and Success Stories

Several case studies have demonstrated the successful implementation of data mining in reproductive health and have led to positive outcomes and impacts.

1.6.1 Utilizing Data Mining for Predicting Reproductive Outcomes Post-Varicocele Embolization

Conducted over a decade, this investigation analyzed information from 293 willing couples undergoing infertility treatments through male varicocele embolization. Employing various data mining techniques including classification, clustering, and association, the researchers assessed factors impacting reproductive outcomes. The study revealed that factors beyond initial sperm parameters, such as the female partner's age, varicocele grade, and exposure to potentially harmful occupational conditions, are correlated with reproductive outcomes. The insights gained from this study contribute to an improved understanding of influencing factors in reproductive outcomes, offering valuable guidance for future treatments (Sousa et al. 2021).

1.6.2 Policy and Practice on Reproductive Health in Brazil, India, Morocco, and Uganda

This paper provides case studies of four countries that analyze how the 1994 International Conference on Population and Development (ICPD) program of action is being implemented. The researchers gathered information through a range of techniques, including data evaluations, interviews with policymakers and healthcare practitioners, and focus group talks with users of reproductive health services. The case studies shed light on changes in reproductive health policies and services, as well as the resources required to support them (1999).

1.6.3 "Nevertheless, You Are Not the First Woman"

Examining Contextual Risk Factors Impacting Sexual and Reproductive Health and Rights in Nicaragua—This case study narrates the experiences of a 19-year-old Nicaraguan woman who faced sexual assault, subsequent pregnancy, and severe complications that almost led to her death. The report identifies violence, unintended pregnancies, and abortion as contextual risk factors influencing sexual and reproductive health and rights in Nicaragua. Analyzing individual women's stories provides insights into contextual risk factors and missed opportunities for enhancing reproductive health and rights (Luffy et al. 2019).

1.6.4 Rita's Data-Driven Approach to Women's Fertility

This experiment began with a survey to collect information on numerous aspects that may affect fertility, such as sleep, water intake, period cycle duration, and others. The team created a set of tools and an app to assist academics in visualizing data from USAID's DHS program, which collects data on health habits from over 80 nations. The goal is to develop a better tool for mining survey data and uncovering trends that will lead to a better understanding of reproductive health (2016).

1.6.5 Big Data for Reproductive Health

For this project, a group of students created a set of tools and an app to assist academics in visualizing data from USAID's DHS program. Based on the summer's Data+ effort, the machine learning tool may forecast a woman's anticipated contraceptive trajectory based on parameters such as age, education level, distance from a clinic, and others. The project's goal is to give people with relevant information while also informing ongoing debates around data collection and contraceptive calendar data (2024).

1.7 Future Directions

Innovative technologies in data mining encompass sophisticated algorithms, machine learning techniques, and big data analytics, sparking a revolution across diverse industries like healthcare, education, and marketing. Some of the pivotal emerging technologies are the following.

1.7.1 Deep Learning

A subset of machine learning that employs artificial neural networks to replicate the learning processes of the human brain. Its applications span diverse domains such as image recognition, natural language processing, and healthcare diagnostics (Lundberg 2023).

1.7.2 Big Data Analytics

The utilization of advanced algorithms and techniques to analyze extensive datasets, unveiling patterns and trends that guide decision-making. Big data analytics finds applications across various sectors, including healthcare, finance, and education (Luan et al. 2020). IoT (Internet of Things): The interconnection of devices and sensors that enable data collection and exchange. IoT has applications in various domains, such as healthcare, manufacturing, and transportation (Lundberg 2023). Emerging technologies in data mining have the potential to improve reproductive health by enabling better analysis of medical data, predicting health outcomes, and optimizing treatment plans. Some potential applications include predicting fertility—By analyzing medical data, researchers can develop models that predict fertility levels in men and women, helping couples plan their families and improve reproductive health outcomes, personalized medicine. Harnessing big data and machine learning methodologies, healthcare providers can formulate personalized treatment plans for patients, considering their medical history, lifestyle, and other factors impacting health outcomes and the early detection of diseases. Advanced algorithms have the capability to scrutinize medical data, recognizing early indicators of reproductive health issues, enabling timely intervention and enhancing patient outcomes.

In the realm of data mining and reproductive health research, numerous research gaps exist. Some of these gaps encompass:

(i) **Data privacy and security:** As medical data is collected and analyzed, privacy and security are concerned. Researchers need to develop methods to protect sensitive information and ensure that data are treated responsibly.
(ii) **Algorithm bias and fairness:** Large-scale data and machine learning algorithms can be influenced by underlying data biases. Researchers need to develop methods for identifying and combating these prejudices in order to ensure that algorithms are fair and accurate for all users.

The amalgamation of Big Data and Artificial Intelligence in education has become a reality, propelled by the swift advancement of technology across various industries. Researchers should examine the potential advantages and disadvantages of applying these technologies in the educational context (Luan et al. 2020).

1.8 Conclusion

In conclusion, this chapter has explored the crucial intersection of reproductive health and data mining, with a specific focus on the potential of machine learning in overcoming challenges within this domain. Reproductive health, encompassing physical, mental, and social well-being, plays a pivotal role in individuals' overall health and quality of life. The incorporation of data mining techniques, encompassing classification, clustering, association rules, and prediction, has surfaced as a transformative influence in tackling the intricacies of reproductive health research.

The chapter highlighted the growing significance of data in healthcare decision-making, emphasizing the role of comprehensive patient health histories in formulating effective treatment plans. As the healthcare industry generates an ever-increasing volume of data, traditional methods become insufficient, paving the way for the adoption of advanced technologies like machine learning to process and analyze vast datasets. The potential impact of data mining in reproductive health research is underscored by its ability to unravel complex relationships within large medical datasets, where traditional statistical methods may fall short. The objectives of the chapter were to provide an in-depth understanding of the basics of data mining, its relevance in healthcare, and its application in the intricate domain of reproductive health. Through exploring the fundamental concepts of data mining, the chapter laid the groundwork for comprehending the transformative potential of machine learning in overcoming traditional research limitations. Real-world applications of data mining in reproductive health, including the utilization of electronic health records, predictive analytics, and disease surveillance, were discussed. These applications demonstrated how data mining techniques could enhance patient care, inform public health policies, and contribute to predictive modelling for reproductive outcomes.

However, challenges and ethical considerations were not overlooked. Concerns related to data quality, accessibility, and privacy were discussed in the context of the increasing interest of for-profit entities in healthcare databases. The chapter emphasized the need for a nuanced approach to address these challenges, considering the delicate nature of reproductive health data. Case studies and success stories provided tangible evidence of the positive impacts of data mining in reproductive health, ranging from predicting reproductive outcomes to informing policy and practice. These examples illustrated the diverse applications and the potential for data mining to contribute to improved reproductive health services globally. Looking forward, emerging technologies such as deep learning, big data analysis, and the Internet of Things (IoT) have been highlighted as transforming forces in the field of data mining. These technologies have the potential to revolutionize reproductive health research by enabling better analysis of medical data, personalized medicine, and early detection of diseases.

In summary, the chapter has laid a comprehensive foundation for understanding the current landscape, challenges, and future directions of data mining in reproductive health. The implications for the future of reproductive health and data mining are vast, promising advancements in personalized medicine, improved patient outcomes, and informed public health policies. As the field continues to evolve, the integration of ethical considerations, privacy safeguards, and responsible data handling practices will be essential to ensure the responsible and beneficial application of data mining techniques in the realm of reproductive health.

Acknowledgments The authors would like to acknowledge the use of AI-based tools such as Quillbot and Grammarly to improve readability and summarize some parts of the text. The authors have further reviewed the text and take full responsibility for the text.

References

Alfawzan N, Christen M, Spitale G, Biller-Andorno N (2022) Privacy, data sharing, and data security policies of women's mHealth apps: scoping review and content analysis. JMIR Mhealth Uhealth 10:e33735. https://doi.org/10.2196/33735

Birjandi SM, Khasteh SH (2021) A survey on data mining techniques used in medicine. J Diabetes Metab Disord 20:2055–2071. https://doi.org/10.1007/s40200-021-00884-2

Bower JK, Bollinger CE, Foraker RE et al (2017) Active use of Electronic Health Records (EHRs) and Personal Health Records (PHRs) for epidemiologic research: sample representativeness and nonresponse bias in a study of women during pregnancy. eGEMs 5:1. https://doi.org/10.13063/2327-9214.1263

Chiruvella V, Guddati AK (2021) Ethical issues in patient data ownership. Interact J Med Res 10:e22269. https://doi.org/10.2196/22269

Dong T, Zhu M, Li R, Wang X (2022) Challenges of utilizing medical big data in reproductive health research. Front Reprod Health 4:800760. https://doi.org/10.3389/frph.2022.800760

Han J, Pei J (2012) Data mining: concepts and techniques. Elsevier

Khanna RR, Murray SG, Wen T et al (2022) Protecting reproductive health information in the post-Roe era: interoperability strategies for healthcare institutions. J Am Med Inform Assoc 30:161–166. https://doi.org/10.1093/jamia/ocac194

Luan H, Geczy P, Lai H et al (2020) Challenges and future directions of big data and artificial intelligence in education. Front Psychol 11:580820. https://doi.org/10.3389/fpsyg.2020.580820

Luffy SM, Evans DP, Rochat RW (2019) "Regardless, you are not the first woman": an illustrative case study of contextual risk factors impacting sexual and reproductive health and rights in Nicaragua. BMC Womens Health 19:76. https://doi.org/10.1186/s12905-019-0771-9

Lundberg L (2023) Bibliometric mining of research directions and trends for big data. J Big Data 10:112. https://doi.org/10.1186/s40537-023-00793-6

Minewiskan (2023) Data mining algorithms (analysis services—data mining). https://learn.microsoft.com/en-us/analysis-services/data-mining/data-mining-algorithms-analysis-services-data-mining?view=asallproducts-allversions

PrognoCIS EHR (2024) The role and importance of data collection in healthcare. In: PrognoCIS EHR. https://prognocis.com/importance-of-data-collection-in-healthcare/

Santos-Pereira J, Gruenwald L, Bernardino J (2022) Top data mining tools for the healthcare industry. J King Saud Univ Comput Inform Sci 34:4968–4982. https://doi.org/10.1016/j.jksuci.2021.06.002

Sousa AP, Santos-Pereira J, Freire MJ et al (2021) Using data mining to assist in predicting reproductive outcomes following varicocele embolization. JCM 10:3503. https://doi.org/10.3390/jcm10163503

Twin A (2003) What is data mining? How it works, benefits, techniques, and examples. In: Investopedia, what is data mining? How it works, benefits, techniques, and examples. https://www.investopedia.com/terms/d/datamining.asp

WHO (2021) Reproductive health, World Health Organization. In: World Health Organization. https://www.who.int/southeastasia/health-topics/reproductive-health. Accessed 12 Mar 2024

Reproductive Health Data Sources

2

Bharati Pandey and Lakshmi Sonkusale

Abstract

Reproductive health data sources are an important step towards the enhancement of research endeavors in the field of reproductive disorders. This chapter overviews the various resources available across the public platforms which are critical for data-driven decision-making and for the policymaker's introduction of effective measures in the evolving healthcare interventions. In the following text, several aspects of data types relevant to reproductive health are discussed such as clinical data, genomic data, and epidemiology data. Further, the chapter delves into the classification of reproductive health data resources based on several criteria, such as the type of organization, the scope of data coverage, and the geographic focus. The chapter also underlines the engagement of public and private organizations and mass initiatives in curating and circulating reproductive health data. One of the key highlights of the chapter is the emphasis on the ethical considerations of aspects of data collection, storage, and sharing, emphasizing the significance of privacy and informed consent in preserving the integrity of sensitive reproductive health information. In the last section, the chapter discusses the various case studies wherein the ethical use of reproductive health data has led to successful implementations of programs and research across different countries.

Keywords

Reproductive health · Telemedicine · eHealth · Fertility · Family planning

B. Pandey (✉) · L. Sonkusale
ICAR-National Dairy Research Institute (NDRI), Karnal, Haryana, India
e-mail: bharti.pandey@icar.gov.in

A. Sengupta et al. (eds.), *Data-Driven Reproductive Health*,
https://doi.org/10.1007/978-981-97-7451-7_2

2.1 Introduction

Reproductive health data play an important role in shaping public health policies and interventions, offering indispensable insights for policymakers, healthcare professionals, and public health organizations. This data is crucial in comprehending, monitoring, and addressing diverse facets of reproductive health. Undoubtedly, reproductive health stands as a fundamental pillar for the social and economic development of communities and nations, representing a core element in human development (World Health Organization 2004). In the context of public health, reproductive health data is foundational for evidence-based policymaking and the successful implementation of public health interventions. It provides essential insights for policymakers, aiding in their understanding of prevalent reproductive health issues, the effectiveness of existing programs, and areas requiring attention and enhancement. Furthermore, this data is instrumental in disease prevention and control, supporting the development of targeted interventions, awareness campaigns, and vaccination programs to mitigate the incidence of reproductive health-related illnesses, particularly sexually transmitted infections. Crucially, reproductive health data plays a pivotal role in monitoring and improving maternal and child health outcomes, guiding interventions based on information about maternal mortality rates, antenatal care utilization, and birth outcomes. Additionally, it is indispensable for the design and evaluation of family planning programs, informing policies to ensure access to various contraceptive methods and supporting initiatives in family planning. Reproductive health data also contributes to identifying disparities in healthcare access, enabling policymakers to implement tailored interventions to address health inequities. Furthermore, the efficient allocation of resources is facilitated through the use of this data, allowing authorities to direct funds, personnel, and infrastructure to areas with higher reproductive health needs. The prevention of maternal mortality is another critical aspect, with data on mortality rates and causes guiding the development of strategies, such as ensuring access to skilled birth attendants and emergency obstetric care. Reproductive health data is a key driver of public awareness and education campaigns, shaping targeted initiatives to promote healthy behaviors and reduce risky practices. Continuous monitoring and evaluation of this data contribute to program assessment and improvement, allowing policymakers to identify successful strategies and areas in need of enhancement, thereby fostering more effective public health initiatives. Lastly, at the global level, reproductive health data facilitates international collaboration and advocacy, enabling organizations and policymakers to comprehend the global landscape, identify shared challenges, and collaboratively implement evidence-based interventions. In conclusion, reproductive health data serves as the linchpin for evidence-based policymaking, guiding effective public health interventions that not only address current challenges but also shape strategies to enhance reproductive health outcomes for individuals and communities. Measuring reproductive health poses challenges, requiring increased awareness among data collectors and users. Determining the effectiveness of reproductive health interventions is inherently difficult. While reproductive health should not receive special pleading for resources, it also should not demand unique standards of proof not met by other healthcare priorities (Graham 1998).

The scope and purpose of reproductive health data sources are extensive and critical for informed decision-making and public health planning. These sources serve as invaluable tools in comprehending, tracking, and enhancing various facets of reproductive health. In terms of scope, they cover a wide range of areas, including fertility and birth rates, where the data helps in deciphering population dynamics and trends. Maternal health indicators, such as mortality rates and antenatal care utilization, are monitored to assess the well-being of pregnant women. Family planning and contraceptive use data track the prevalence of methods, ensuring informed family planning programs. Information on sexually transmitted infections (STIs) aids in guiding prevention and treatment strategies, while a focus on adolescent reproductive health addresses the unique needs of this demographic. Abortion data collection informs policies, and data on gender-based violence sheds light on intimate partner violence and sexual violence. Exploring infertility, reproductive technologies, and the utilization of reproductive health services further enriches the scope. Additionally, demographic and population trends analysis allow for a comprehensive understanding of population structures.

2.2 Types of Reproductive Datasets

Introduction to the various types of reproductive datasets utilized in research and clinical practice encompasses a range of crucial data sources. These include clinical data, which involves detailed information obtained during patient care, genomic data that delves into the genetic aspects of reproduction, imaging data providing visual insights, and epidemiological data, which aids in understanding the patterns and determinants of reproductive health on a broader scale. The integration of these diverse datasets plays a vital role in advancing our understanding of reproductive processes and enhancing both research and clinical interventions in this field. The field of reproductive health research and clinical practice relies on a diverse array of datasets to unravel the complexities of human reproduction. These datasets can be broadly categorized into clinical data, genomic data, imaging data, and epidemiological data, each offering unique insights into various facets of reproductive health.

2.3 Clinical Data

It is the backbone of reproductive health research, encompassing information derived from medical records, patient histories, and laboratory results. This data includes details on fertility treatments, pregnancy outcomes, and maternal health, providing a comprehensive understanding of individual patient experiences and healthcare outcomes. Hospital-based case-control studies are often deemed more reliable in providing information on medical conditions compared to their population-based counterparts. This increased reliability stems from the shared setting, ensuring similar attention to the medical history of both cases and controls within the hospital environment. Despite this advantage, criticisms have arisen. Concerns revolve around potential associations between the factors being studied and the admission diseases of controls, raising questions about the validity of the data collected. Additionally, there is a recognition of potential substantial differences between information gathered within the hospital setting and that obtained outside of it (Bosetti et al. 2001). These critiques highlight the need for a nuanced interpretation of findings from hospital-based case-control studies, considering the intricate relationships between study factors, admission diseases, and the context in which information is collected.

2.4 Genomic Data

Genomic data is invaluable in shaping our understanding of reproductive health, guiding personalized interventions, and advancing the field of reproductive medicine. It empowers individuals and healthcare professionals with information to make informed decisions regarding family planning and fertility treatments. It refers to the information encoded in an organism's DNA, which includes the complete set of genes and non-coding sequences. It can be analyzed to understand the genetic makeup of an individual, population, or species. Several challenges in genomics from the essential informatics requirements for storing and analyzing raw sequencing data generated by highly multiplexed sequencing technologies. In the current landscape, a single week-long sequencing run can yield data volumes equivalent to those produced by entire genome centers just a few years ago. It has become standard practice for many laboratories engaged in genomic research to grapple with the imperative of handling terabytes of information. The existence of extensive and sizable genomic datasets gives rise to concerns regarding information access, data security, and the privacy of subjects/patients. Addressing these concerns requires careful consideration to ensure the continued rapid progress of the field (Kahn 2011).

2.5 Image Data

Image data refers to information represented in the form of visual images. These images can be in various formats, such as JPEG, PNG, GIF, or others, and they are composed of pixels arranged in a grid. Image data is widely used in different fields, including computer vision, medical imaging, satellite imagery, photography, and more. It plays a crucial role in reproductive health, particularly in fields like obstetrics and gynecology. Ultrasound, magnetic resonance imaging (MRI), and other imaging techniques provide detailed visualizations of reproductive organs, aiding in the diagnosis of conditions such as infertility, pregnancy complications, and reproductive tract abnormalities. Modern medical imaging technologies now generate images at the cellular level, leading to the increased visibility of egg and sperm cells, which have consequently become well-known elements in popular culture. This transformation is a result of medical imaging technologies turning these gametes from invisible components integrated into biological processes within the body into recognizable objects. The visualization of egg and sperm cells has essentially removed the process of human reproduction from the confines of the female body, casting the gametes as central figures in the narrative of human reproduction (Lie 2015).

2.6 Epidemiological Data

Epidemiological data are crucial for identifying patterns of diseases, understanding their causes, and informing public health policies and interventions. Researchers and public health professionals use these data to assess the impact of diseases on populations, identify trends over time, and develop strategies for disease prevention and control. Gathering accurate and comprehensive epidemiological data is essential for making informed decisions aimed at improving the overall health and well-being of communities (Taskinen 1993). The integration of these diverse datasets allows researchers and clinicians to take a comprehensive and multidimensional approach to reproductive health, fostering a deeper understanding of the intricate interplay between genetic, clinical, imaging, and population-level factors in the realm of human reproduction. Epidemiological data were collected to assess potential risks associated with exposure to static and time-varying magnetic fields utilized in magnetic resonance (MR) imaging (Kanal et al. 1993).

2.7 Data Sources

Access to reproductive health data is essential for researchers, policymakers, healthcare professionals, and organizations working to improve reproductive health outcomes. Reproductive health data resources can be classified based on various criteria, including the type of organization, the scope of data coverage, and the geographic focus. National reproductive health data sources vary by country, and each country typically has its institutions and agencies responsible for collecting and disseminating reproductive health information. Some common types of national reproductive health data sources are as follows.

2.7.1 National Statistical Offices

Most countries have a national statistical office or agency responsible for collecting and disseminating demographic and health-related data. These offices often conduct national censuses and surveys that include modules on reproductive health.

2.7.2 Ministries of Health

The Ministry of Health or equivalent government department is a key player in collecting and managing health data, including reproductive health indicators. They may conduct surveys, maintain health registries, and oversee health information systems.

2.7.3 National Health Surveys

Many countries conduct periodic national health surveys that include specific modules on reproductive health. Examples include the Demographic and Health Surveys (DHS), Reproductive Health Surveys, and Maternal and Child Health Surveys.

2.7.4 Vital Registration Systems

Vital registration systems, managed by government agencies, record vital events such as births, deaths, and marriages. These systems provide essential data for monitoring reproductive health, including fertility rates and maternal mortality.

2.7.5 Health Information Systems

Countries often have health information systems that collect and manage data from healthcare facilities. These systems can provide information on maternal health services, family planning, and other reproductive health-related services.

2.7.6 National Family Planning Programs

Programs focused on family planning and reproductive health may maintain data on contraceptive use, family planning services, and related indicators. These programs are often run by government health agencies or in collaboration with NGOs.

2.7.7 National Institutes of Health

Some countries have specific institutes or research bodies dedicated to health research. These institutions may conduct studies and research projects related to reproductive health and contribute valuable data.

2.7.8 Reproductive Health Surveys and Studies

Governments or research organizations may conduct specific reproductive health surveys and studies to gather detailed information on issues such as fertility, contraception, maternal health, and sexually transmitted infections.

2.7.9 Maternal and Child Health Programs

Programs focused on maternal and child health often collect and maintain data on maternal health outcomes, antenatal care, childbirth, and postnatal care.

When accessing national reproductive health data, it is important to check the specific sources relevant to each country. These sources may collaborate with international organizations, such as the World Health Organization (WHO) and the United Nations Population Fund (UNFPA), to ensure standardized data collection and reporting practices. International reproductive health data sources provide a global perspective on various aspects of reproductive health. These sources often collect, analyze, and disseminate data from multiple countries, allowing for cross-country comparisons and the identification of global trends. Some key international reproductive health data sources are as follows:

(i) **World Health Organization (WHO):** The WHO is a major international organization that collects and publishes global health data, including reproductive health indicators. The Global Health Observatory (GHO) is a valuable resource for accessing WHO's reproductive health statistics.

(ii) **United Nations Population Fund (UNFPA):** UNFPA focuses on issues related to population and reproductive health at the global level. It provides data, reports, and support programs to improve reproductive health worldwide.

(iii) **World Bank:** The World Bank collects and publishes global economic and social data, including reproductive health indicators. The World Development Indicators (WDI) database is a comprehensive source for global health data.

(iv) **Demographic and Health Surveys (DHS):** The DHS program conducts surveys in numerous countries to collect demographic and health data, including reproductive health indicators. It provides standardized and comparable datasets for cross-country analyses.

(v) **Guttmacher Institute:** The Guttmacher Institute is a research organization that focuses on sexual and reproductive health globally. It conducts studies, research, and publishes reports on topics such as family planning, abortion, and adolescent sexual health.
(vi) **UNICEF:** The United Nations Children's Fund (UNICEF) provides data on maternal and child health, including indicators related to reproductive health. The State of the World's Children and other reports include relevant information.
(vii) **Population Reference Bureau (PRB):** PRB is a non-profit organization that provides demographic data and analysis at the global level. It produces reports on population trends, reproductive health, and related topics.
(viii) **International Planned Parenthood Federation (IPPF):** IPPF is a global organization that works on sexual and reproductive health and rights. They provide data and reports on family planning, contraception, and related issues.
(ix) **United Nations Statistics Division (UNSD):** UNSD compiles and disseminates global statistical information, including demographic and health data. It collaborates with various organizations to maintain international statistical standards.
(x) **Reproductive Health Global Partnerships:** Global partnerships and initiatives, such as the Family Planning 2020 (FP2020) and Every Woman Every Child, work towards improving reproductive health outcomes globally. They often provide data and progress reports.
(xi) **International Health Organizations:** Organizations like the International Planned Parenthood Federation (IPPF), Médecins Sans Frontières (Doctors Without Borders), and others contribute to global reproductive health efforts and may provide relevant data.

2.8 Case Studies: A Few Examples of Successful Reproductive Health Data Utilization

2.8.1 Family Planning in Rwanda

In Rwanda, a significant challenge in family planning programs is the high discontinuation rate, with almost a third of contraceptive users stopping within the first year. This qualitative study conducted between February and July 2018 explores strategies employed by family planning providers and contraceptive users to address this issue. Providers focus on counseling, reminders, and support for dissatisfied users, while users emphasize understanding side effects, peer support, persistence, and method switching. These strategies indicate the potential for long-term sustained contraception use in Rwanda, emphasizing the importance of supporting and harnessing such approaches for continued success in family planning programs (Schwandt et al. 2021).

2.8.2 HIV Prevention in Thailand

Against the backdrop of a heightened prevalence of HIV/AIDS, especially within key populations, Thailand grappled with the imperative to curb the epidemic's spread. To tackle this pressing issue, the government harnessed data obtained from HIV surveillance programs and clinical records to pinpoint high-risk groups and geographical areas. Armed with this insightful information, the country executed a comprehensive set of targeted prevention strategies. These included widespread educational campaigns, the distribution of condoms, and community-based interventions tailored to address the specific needs of identified high-risk groups. The impact of these data-driven interventions was notable, contributing significantly to the reduction of HIV transmission rates across the nation. This success underscored the pivotal role that data utilization plays in the development and implementation of effective public health strategies, especially in the context of combating infectious diseases and safeguarding the health of vulnerable populations.

Explores the historical development of three prominent HIV/AIDS initiatives in Thailand: a civil society campaign promoting condom usage, the Ministry of Public Health's 100% condom program targeting high-risk populations, and a universal Prevention of Mother-To-Child Transmission (PMTCT) program. Using a comparative and historical approach, the study identifies common factors contributing to the success of these initiatives, including dedicated policy entrepreneurs, successful demonstration projects establishing credible evidence, and collaboration with diverse institutional partners. The findings emphasize the crucial role of demonstration projects in policy adoption and the impact of diverse partnerships in scaling initiatives nationally. The analysis highlights the evolution of these programs from vertical to integrated approaches, mirroring global changes in the HIV/AIDS landscape (Harris and Thaiprayoon 2022).

2.8.3 Teen Pregnancy Prevention in the United States

In the United States, the pervasive issue of high teen pregnancy rates poses significant social and economic challenges. To address this concern, the nation turned to comprehensive data gathered through national surveys, notably the Youth Risk Behavior Surveillance System (YRBSS), which systematically documented risky behaviors, including rates of sexual activity among teenagers. Armed with this crucial data, policymakers and public health officials strategically devised comprehensive sex education programs and community outreach initiatives tailored to the specific needs and challenges identified. Over time, the impact of these interventions became evident as the nation witnessed a notable decline in teen pregnancy rates. This success story highlights the instrumental role that data utilization plays in crafting targeted interventions, ultimately contributing to positive shifts in societal trends and improved reproductive health outcomes.

Efforts to combat adolescent pregnancy in the United States involve a review of prevention strategies, emphasizing lessons learned and future directions. Despite reductions, disparities persist based on race, geography, and socioeconomic status. Current programs often fall short, leaving many adolescents underserved. Addressing these challenges requires considering social determinants of health, structural racism, and promoting equity and inclusion. Recommendations include improving education programs, involving youth in policy design, using technology for health literacy, expanding access through telehealth, and creating inclusive policies that confront structural racism and prioritize health equity (Brindis et al. 2020).

2.8.4 Maternal Health in India

In India, the persistent challenge of maternal mortality, particularly prevalent in rural areas with constrained access to healthcare, prompted a strategic response from the government. Leveraging data sourced from health records and maternal health surveys, the government undertook a comprehensive analysis to identify regions with elevated risks and ascertain the factors contributing to maternal deaths. Informed by this critical information, targeted interventions were deployed, including the establishment of mobile health clinics and the mobilization of community health workers to address healthcare gaps in these identified high-risk areas. The impact of these data-driven initiatives was substantial, reflected in a notable decrease in maternal mortality rates within the targeted regions. This success underscores the transformative potential of utilizing health data to inform and guide precise interventions, thereby fostering positive changes in maternal health outcomes and narrowing the healthcare disparity gap in underserved regions.

India, a significant contributor to global maternal deaths, aims to reduce maternal mortality to less than 100 per 100,000 live births. Despite economic progress and programmatic efforts, achieving this goal remains distant. The vast geography and sociocultural diversity lead to varying maternal mortality rates across states, hindering uniform health-sector reforms. This case study examines national maternal mortality trends, healthcare delivery systems, and program implementation. It highlights challenges, such as limited success and proposes solutions: improved reporting, evidence-based strategies, effective monitoring, private sector regulation, increased public-private partnerships, and strengthened political will and management capacity to enhance maternal health (Vora et al. 2009).

2.8.5 Adolescent Reproductive Health in Ethiopia

In Ethiopia, the prevalent challenges of early marriage and adolescent pregnancies compelled the government to address these issues through a data-driven approach. Harnessing data obtained from household surveys and community-based research, the government gained valuable insights into the factors contributing to the high rates of early marriages and pregnancies among adolescents. Armed with this knowledge, policymakers adjusted existing policies, and community-led initiatives were strategically implemented to raise awareness about the significance of education and the importance of delaying marriage. These targeted interventions, guided by the wealth of data, played a pivotal role in contributing to a substantial decline in adolescent pregnancies across the country. This success story underscores the transformative impact of utilizing data to inform policy decisions and implement community-driven initiatives, thereby positively influencing societal norms and fostering improved reproductive health outcomes among Ethiopia's adolescent population.

This article addresses the lack of evidence on early adolescent perspectives on sexual and reproductive health (SRH) in Ethiopia and Rwanda. Drawing from a qualitative research study with 10- to 12-year-olds and 14- to 15-year-olds, it uses Amartya Sen's capability approach. Focusing on SRH, the article examines the influence of gendered social norms on adolescents' experiences, revealing three key themes: puberty transitions, sexuality, and victim blaming. The study emphasizes the impact of discriminatory social norms on health service uptake, concluding with a call to strategically address these norms to support young people in navigating their sexual and reproductive lives (Coast et al. 2019).

Reproductive health data can be obtained from a variety of sources, each offering a unique perspective on different aspects of reproductive health. Figure 2.1 shows several common sources below. The integration of data from these diverse sources allows for a more comprehensive understanding of reproductive health, enabling policymakers, healthcare providers, and researchers to make informed decisions and implement effective interventions. However, challenges such as data quality, privacy, and representativeness should be addressed to ensure the reliability and usefulness of the collected information.

2.9 Mobile App and Web App for Human Reproductive Data in India

Some general categories of apps related to reproductive health and wellness are given in Table 2.1. The table presents data related to a mobile app designed for collecting and managing human reproductive data in India. The app aims to address

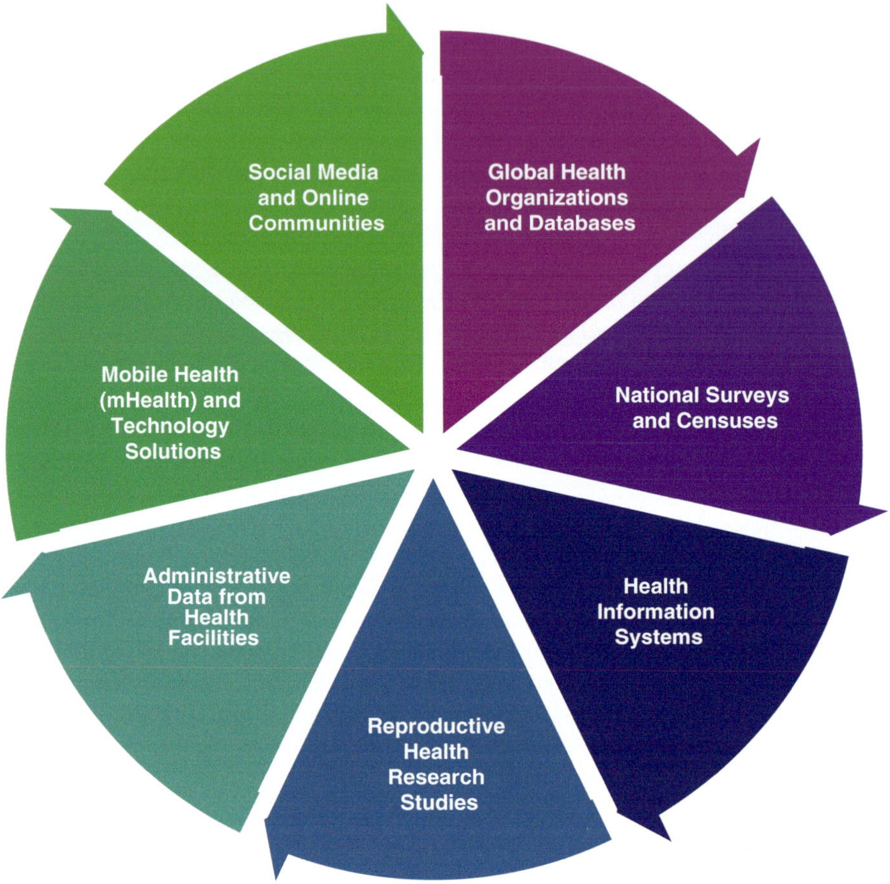

Fig. 2.1 Snapshot of reproductive data sources

various aspects of reproductive health and provide a platform for users to track and access relevant information. Table 2.2 tells the online web pages or web apps related to reproductive health.

2.10 Challenges in Reproductive Health Data Collection

Challenges in reproductive health data collection can arise from various factors, including cultural, logistical, ethical, and technical considerations. Here are some common challenges associated with collecting reproductive health data (Wasserheit and Holmes 1992; Gyimah et al. 2006).

Table 2.1 Mobile app for human reproductive data in India

S.N.	Mobile apps	Purpose	Accessible links
1.	• Clue • Glow • Flo • MyDays • Natural Cycles • Oura Period Prediction • Ovia Fertility	Period tracking and fertility	https://play.google.com/store/apps/details?id=com.clue.android&hl=en_GB&pli=1 https://www.womenshealthmag.com/health/g26787041/best-period-tracking-apps/ https://www.healthline.com/health/pregnancy/fertility-apps#our-picks
2.	• BabyCenter • What to Expect • Ovia Pregnancy Tracker • Pregnancy Tracker & Countdown to Baby Due Date • Amila • Glow Nurture • WeMoms • Baby Bump • Preglife.	Pregnancy and maternity	https://www.noodleandboo.com/blogs/journal/best-pregnancy-apps-for-tracking-your-babys-development https://preglife.com/ https://www.wemoms.com/ https://www.thebump.com/ https://www.babycenter.com/pregnancy https://www.whattoexpect.com/mobile-app/
3.	• Fitbit (includes menstrual cycle tracking) • Apple Health (includes reproductive health tracking) • Google Fit	Health and wellness	https://tipalti.com/guide/best-wellness-apps-2023/
4.	• Practo • DocsApp • MFine • 1 mg (health and medicine app) • Lemonaid	Telemedicine	https://www.plumhq.com/blog/the-best-telemedicine-apps-in-india https://getstream.io/blog/best-telemedicine-apps/
5.	• Pink Parcel • Maya (Period, Fertility, Ovulation & Pregnancy) • Women's Health Mag • femtech	Women's health and reproductive education	https://shakuro.com/blog/womens-health-app-blueprint

Table 2.2 Web portals for human reproductive data

Web Apps/Web page	Purpose	Accessible links
data.world	Providing reproductive health data	https://data.world/datasets/reproductive-health
Maternal mortality	Data-related maternal mortality	https://data.unicef.org/topic/maternal-health/maternal-mortality/
USAID	Family planning and reproductive health	https://www.usaid.gov/global-health/health-areas/family-planning

(continued)

Table 2.2 (continued)

Web Apps/Web page	Purpose	Accessible links
SRHAD	Sexual and reproductive health activity dataset collection	https://digital.nhs.uk/data-and-information/data-collections-and-data-sets/data-collections/sexual-and-reproductive-health-activity-data-set-srhad-collection
DataBank	Exploring databases of reproductive health	https://databank.worldbank.org/databases/reproductive-health
HRP	Sexual and reproductive health and rights	https://www.who.int/teams/sexual-and-reproductive-health-and-research-(srh)/human-reproduction-programme
Guttmacher	Good reproductive health	https://www.guttmacher.org/

2.10.1 Stigma and Sensitivity

Reproductive health issues, such as family planning, sexually transmitted infections, and abortion, are often surrounded by stigma. This stigma can lead to underreporting and reluctance to participate in data collection efforts.

2.10.2 Cultural and Societal Norms

Cultural beliefs and societal norms may influence the willingness of individuals to disclose sensitive information related to reproductive health. Privacy concerns and fear of judgment may deter accurate reporting.

2.10.3 Incomplete or Inaccurate Reporting

Individuals may provide incomplete or inaccurate information due to recall bias, social desirability bias, or a lack of understanding of the questions being asked. This can compromise the reliability of the collected data.

2.10.4 Access to Healthcare Services

Disparities in access to healthcare services may result in uneven representation in data. People with limited access to healthcare facilities, particularly in rural or underserved areas, may be underrepresented in reproductive health data.

2.10.5 Data Quality and Standardization

Inconsistent data quality standards across different regions or healthcare facilities can pose challenges in aggregating and comparing reproductive health data. Lack of standardization may hinder the interoperability of data systems.

2.10.6 Resource Constraints

Limited resources, both financial and human, can impact the scope and scale of data collection efforts. This may lead to inadequate sample sizes, incomplete datasets, and challenges in maintaining long-term surveillance.

2.10.7 Technological Barriers

Some regions may face challenges in adopting and implementing advanced data collection technologies. This includes issues related to the availability of infrastructure, Internet connectivity, and the digital divide in certain populations.

2.10.8 Ethical Considerations

Ensuring ethical practices in reproductive health data collection is crucial. Researchers must navigate issues such as informed consent, confidentiality, and the potential harm associated with collecting and sharing sensitive information.

2.10.9 Longitudinal Challenges

Conducting longitudinal studies in reproductive health requires sustained efforts over an extended period. Attrition rates and participant dropouts can impact the validity of longitudinal data.

2.10.10 Policy and Regulatory Challenges

Inconsistent or inadequate policies and regulations governing the collection, storage, and use of reproductive health data can impede research efforts. Ensuring compliance with ethical standards is essential.

2.10.11 Interdisciplinary Collaboration

Reproductive health data often require collaboration between various disciplines, including healthcare, sociology, and public health. Bridging the gap between these disciplines and fostering effective communication can be challenging.

Addressing these challenges requires a comprehensive and multi-faceted approach, involving careful planning, community engagement, ethical considerations, and the use of innovative technologies. Researchers and policymakers should collaborate to develop strategies that promote accurate, representative, and ethically collected reproductive health data.

2.11 Conclusion

Reproductive health data sources are diverse and continually evolving, reflecting the dynamic nature of the field. Harnessing the full potential of these sources requires ongoing efforts to address challenges related to data quality, privacy, and inclusivity. As technology continues to advance, and new methodologies emerge, the integration of multiple data sources will enhance our ability to monitor and improve reproductive health outcomes, ultimately contributing to the well-being of individuals and communities worldwide. Health is a holistic concept not merely focusing on the absence of disease, but encompassing physical, emotional, and social well-being related to the reproductive system. Its significance resonates in its profound impact on individual rights, public health, gender equality, and the overall development of societies.

Acknowledgments The authors would like to acknowledge the use of AI-based tools such as Quillbot and Grammarly to improve readability and summarize some parts of the text. The authors have further reviewed the text and take full responsibility for the text.

References

Bosetti C, Tavani A, Negri E et al (2001) Reliability of data on medical conditions, menstrual and reproductive history provided by hospital controls. J Clin Epidemiol 54:902–906. https://doi.org/10.1016/S0895-4356(01)00362-6

Brindis CD, Decker MJ, Gutmann-Gonzalez A, Berglas NF (2020) Perspectives on adolescent pregnancy prevention strategies in the United States: looking Back, looking forward. AHMT 11:135–145. https://doi.org/10.2147/AHMT.S219949

Coast E, Jones N, Francoise UM et al (2019) Adolescent sexual and reproductive health in Ethiopia and Rwanda: a qualitative exploration of the role of social norms. SAGE Open 9:215824401983358. https://doi.org/10.1177/2158244019833587

Graham WJ (1998) Outcomes and effectiveness in reproductive health. Soc Sci Med 47:1925–1936. https://doi.org/10.1016/S0277-9536(98)00334-7

Gyimah SO, Takyi BK, Addai I (2006) Challenges to the reproductive-health needs of African women: on religion and maternal health utilization in Ghana. Soc Sci Med 62:2930–2944. https://doi.org/10.1016/j.socscimed.2005.11.034

Harris J, Thaiprayoon S (2022) Common factors in HIV/AIDS prevention success: lessons from Thailand. BMC Health Serv Res 22:1487. https://doi.org/10.1186/s12913-022-08786-6

Kahn SD (2011) On the future of genomic data. Science 331:728–729. https://doi.org/10.1126/science.1197891

Kanal E, Gillen J, Evans JA et al (1993) Survey of reproductive health among female MR workers. Radiology 187:395–399. https://doi.org/10.1148/radiology.187.2.8475280

Lie M (2015) Reproduction inside/outside: medical imaging and the domestication of assisted reproductive technologies. Eur J Women's Stud 22:53–69. https://doi.org/10.1177/1350506814545093

Schwandt H, Boulware A, Corey J et al (2021) Family planning providers and contraceptive users in Rwanda employ strategies to prevent discontinuation. BMC Womens Health 21:361. https://doi.org/10.1186/s12905-021-01503-1

Taskinen HK (1993) Epidemiological studies in monitoring reproductive effects. Environ Health Perspect 101:279–283. https://doi.org/10.1289/ehp.93101s3279

Vora KS, Mavalankar DV, Ramani K et al (2009) Maternal health situation in India: a case study. J Health Popul Nutr 27:184–201. https://doi.org/10.3329/jhpn.v27i2.3363

Wasserheit JN, Holmes KK (1992) Reproductive tract infections: challenges for international health policy, programs, and research. In: Germain A, Holmes KK, Piot P, Wasserheit JN (eds) Reproductive tract infections. Springer US, Boston, pp 7–33

World Health Organization (2004) Measuring access to reproductive health services: Report of a WHO (No. WHO/RHR/04.11). World Health Organization.

Preprocessing and Integration of Reproductive Health Data

3

K. S. Kishor Bharadwaj, Yegna Subramanian Jambunath, Kunal D. Patil, T. J. Ramnath Babu, and D. B. Santosh Bhargav

Abstract

The process of preprocessing and data integration in reproductive health and medicine goes far beyond mere data management. It plays a critical role in enhancing data quality, streamlining operational processes, and leveraging data-driven insights to drive innovations within the field of reproductive medicine. This chapter delves into the digital transformation in clinical care and resource allocation with administrative efficiency to drive groundbreaking research, particularly in the domains of machine learning (ML) and bioinformatics, these ideas have far-reaching impacts that reverberate throughout the landscape of assisted reproductive technology (ART). Further, the chapter discusses the transition of digitization of physical records and the concept of data hub wherein a central platform is fundamental for streamlined data management, report generation, analysis, and research. As an extension to the centralized data hub, a classic example of the ArogyaSetu mobile application during COVID-19 is discussed in detail as a case study. The next section talks about "Why we need an ocean of data in reproductive healthcare considering the challenges and ethical aspects of it." Further it also discusses about data preprocessing the necessity of sanity-checks, standardization, anonymization, normalization, and validation of the data. The next section deals with the challenges in data preprocessing. The last section is about the integration of reproductive health data and shows the dashboard with user interaction and insight visualization. Finally, in a nutshell, the

K. S. Kishor Bharadwaj (✉) · Y. S. Jambunath · K. D. Patil · T. J. Ramnath Babu · D. B. Santosh Bhargav
SpOvum Technologies Private Limited, Bengaluru, India
e-mail: kishor.ks@spovum.com

A. Sengupta et al. (eds.), *Data-Driven Reproductive Health*,
https://doi.org/10.1007/978-981-97-7451-7_3

chapter concludes with the last section, where harnessing the power of data in assisted reproductive technology (ART) is discussed.

Keywords

Digitization · Centralization · Anonymization · Standardization · Visualization Dashboard

3.1 Introduction

Data is the backbone of modern reproductive health research, bridging the gap between clinical observations and scientific breakthroughs. However, raw data is often like an unpolished diamond—full of potential but needing refinement. This chapter delves into the art and science of data preprocessing and integration, crucial steps that transform fragmented, noisy datasets into reliable, actionable insights. Through sophisticated methodologies such as standardization, normalization, and validation, we ensure that the data speaks a language both clinicians and algorithms can understand. But it doesn't end there. As we integrate diverse sources, from patient records to laboratory results, we build comprehensive data ecosystems that fuel innovation in assisted reproductive technology (ART). The aim is not merely to manage data, but to empower it, setting the stage for pioneering research in machine learning and bioinformatics. After all, in the world of reproductive health, a well-preprocessed dataset is like a good match-maker-bringing together all the right variables to create something truly extraordinary.

3.2 Embracing Digital Transformation in Reproductive Health Data Management

3.2.1 Transitioning from Paper to Pixels: The Role of Machine Learning in Data Digitization

In the realm of reproductive health and medicine, the evolution from traditional paper-based records to digital formats represents a significant leap forward. This transition is not merely a change in the medium of data storage; it embodies a paradigm shift in how we approach, manage, and utilize health information. Machine learning (ML), at the forefront of this revolution, serves as a pivotal tool in expediting data entry, enhancing data accuracy, and reinforcing data integrity. Reproductive healthcare encompasses a broad spectrum of medical services related to women's reproductive health, including family planning, pregnancy and childbirth, and gynecological care. Traditionally, the management of reproductive health relied heavily on paper-based records and physician intuition. However, the digital revolution has ushered in a new era, paving the way for data-driven approaches that hold immense potential to revolutionize this critical field.

3.3 Why Data Digitization?

Digitization opens avenues for patient empowerment through increased access to personalized health information. Platforms for patient portals enable secure access to medical records, test results, and educational resources, promoting informed decision-making and shared medical responsibility (Till et al. 2023). Mobile apps can track menstrual cycles, ovulation, and fertility awareness, fostering proactive reproductive health management.

3.3.1 Clinical Precision

Electronic medical records (EMRs) facilitate the storage, retrieval, and analysis of health data, fostering data-driven clinical decision-making (Char et al. 2018). Advanced algorithms can analyze electronic health records to identify patients at risk for specific reproductive health complications, enabling early intervention and preventive measures.

3.3.2 Optimizing Healthcare Delivery

Telemedicine platforms offer virtual consultations with healthcare providers, improving access to care, particularly in underserved areas (Earle et al. 2021). Remote monitoring technologies with wearable devices and biosensors enable real-time tracking of vital signs and fetal well-being, allowing for prompt interventions in pregnancy complications.

3.3.3 Digitizing Historical Records

The journey begins with the digitization of historical health records. Machine learning algorithms, particularly those based on Optical Character Recognition (OCR), have shown remarkable efficacy in converting vast volumes of paper documents into digital data.

3.3.4 Enhancing Data Accuracy

Machine learning also plays a critical role in enhancing the accuracy of the entered data. Traditional manual data entry is prone to human error, often leading to inaccuracies in patient records. ML algorithms, through pattern recognition and error detection capabilities, significantly reduce these errors.

3.3.5 Data Integrity and Security

With digital formats, ensuring data integrity and security becomes paramount. Machine learning algorithms contribute to maintaining the sanctity of data by detecting and preventing unauthorized access or alterations. Advanced ML-based security systems are capable of real-time monitoring of data access, ensuring that the data remains intact and secure from potential breaches.

3.3.6 Visualizing Data Integrity

To illustrate the importance of data integrity, consider a scenario where patient data from various clinics are integrated into a central repository. An ML algorithm could be deployed to continuously monitor the data flow, flagging any inconsistencies or unauthorized changes. A visual representation of this might include a dashboard displaying real-time data flow, with alerts for any detected anomalies. The landscape of reproductive healthcare is undergoing a paradigm shift through the transformative power of data digitization. This section explores the multifaceted significance of digital health solutions in empowering patients, driving clinical precision, and optimizing healthcare delivery. We delve into the potential of patient-generated health data, electronic medical records, and real-time monitoring in enhancing the quality and accessibility of reproductive care. Furthermore, we analyze the ethical considerations and challenges associated with data privacy, security, and equitable access.

3.4 Ethical Considerations and Challenges of Data Digitization

Despite the undeniable benefits, data digitization in reproductive healthcare presents ethical challenges and potential drawbacks.

3.4.1 Privacy and Security

Ensuring the privacy and security of sensitive health data is paramount. Robust data governance frameworks and stringent cybersecurity measures are necessary to prevent unauthorized access and data breaches.

3.4.2 Algorithmic Bias

AI algorithms analyzing health data can perpetuate existing biases based on factors like race, socioeconomic status, and geographic location (Char et al. 2018). Mitigating algorithmic bias through diverse datasets and transparent algorithms is crucial to ensure equitable access to quality healthcare.

3.4.3 Digital Divide

Unequal access to technology and digital literacy can exacerbate existing disparities in healthcare access (Earle et al. 2021). Bridging the digital divide through targeted interventions and promoting digital literacy is essential to ensure inclusive benefits of data digitization.

The digitization of reproductive healthcare presents a unique opportunity to improve the quality, accessibility, and affordability of care. However, navigating the ethical landscape and addressing challenges will be critical to unlocking the full potential of this transformative technology. By emphasizing patient empowerment, data privacy, and inclusive access, we can ensure that data digitization catalyzes achieving equitable and personalized reproductive healthcare for all.

Data digitization in reproductive health research is a pivotal advancement that offers numerous benefits, including enhanced data accessibility, improved data quality, efficient analysis, longitudinal monitoring, and ethical considerations. Embracing these technological advancements is crucial for advancing our understanding of reproductive health and improving outcomes for individuals and communities using mathematical principles.

In the next Sect. B, we see what different mathematical tools are used in the processing of digital data. In this regard, we shall understand the differences between two main mathematical methods one being classical mathematical statistics and another being artificial intelligence-based machine learning.

3.5 Distinction Between ML and Statistics

Machine learning (ML) and statistics are two closely related fields that share foundational principles in data analysis, yet they differ significantly in their objectives, methodologies, and applications. Table 3.1 explores the key distinctions between machine learning and statistics, shedding light on their unique characteristics.

Table 3.1 A comparison between machine learning and statistics

Particulars	Machine learning (ML)	Statistics
Objective and focus	Developing algorithms that enable computers to learn patterns and make predictions or decisions without explicit programming (Hastie et al. 2009).	Traditionally focuses on inference, hypothesis testing, and understanding the underlying processes that generate data (Freedman 2003).
Scope of application	Emphasizes predictive modeling and pattern recognition in diverse applications, including image recognition, natural language processing, and recommendation systems (Bishop 2016).	Broader scope, encompassing experimental design, hypothesis testing, and estimation in economics, biology, and psychology (Wackerly et al. 2008). Statistics is commonly used to conclude populations based on sample data.
Approach to data	Tends to focus on leveraging algorithms to automatically learn patterns and relationships from data, often with an emphasis on model accuracy and generalization to new data (James et al. 2013).	The emphasis is on using data to make inferences about populations, estimating parameters, and testing hypotheses, with a strong foundation in probability theory (Casella and Berger 2002).
Model complexity and interpretability	Machine learning models often embrace high complexity, utilizing intricate algorithms and deep neural networks to capture intricate patterns in data (Goodfellow et al. 2016).	Statistical models, such as linear regression or analysis of variance, are generally more interpretable and are designed to capture specific relationships between variables with a focus on understanding the underlying processes (Fox 2016).
Evolution and adaptability	Machine learning has evolved rapidly in response to the increasing availability of big data and computational power, leading to the development of sophisticated models like deep learning (LeCun et al. 2015).	Statistics has adapted as well, incorporating Bayesian methods and resampling techniques, but tends to have a more traditional foundation in frequentist statistics (Fox 2016).

While machine learning and statistics share common roots in data analysis, their distinct objectives, scopes, approaches to data, model complexities, and adaptabilities mark them as separate but complementary fields. Understanding these distinctions is crucial for researchers and practitioners in both domains to effectively apply the appropriate methods to address specific analytical challenges.

In a nutshell, the transition to digital data management in reproductive health, bolstered by machine learning, is not just a technological upgrade but a fundamental enhancement in the way we handle sensitive health data. This shift promises greater efficiency, accuracy, and security, paving the way for more informed and effective reproductive health care.

In the next Sect. C, we see the significance of digitized data which is available at one place similar to a data lake or a data hub.

3.6 Data Hub

The idea of data collection and integration leads to the "Data Hub" in ART, which serves as a critical platform, aggregating and structuring data from a wide array of sources. The sources include but are not limited to, double witnessing systems, computer-aided semen analysis (CASA) systems, lab parameters monitoring, and alarming systems, embryo monitoring systems (EMS), programmable ICSI manipulators (Bharadwaj et al. 2022), other novel electronic micromanipulation technologies such as those for manipulating oocytes and embryos, automated data collection systems, metadata recording tools, and various forms of human input data. By collating this diverse range of information, the data hub plays an essential role in the effective management of data, facilitating the generation of detailed reports, thorough analysis, and supporting research in reproductive medicine. This comprehensive approach to data integration is pivotal for deriving meaningful insights and aiding in informed decision-making in the field. The data centralization hub can be effectively achieved through a dual-method approach to data collection, encompassing both local data collection and central data collection. Each method plays a distinct yet complementary role in the overall data management and analysis process.

3.7 Local Data Collection

At the local level, individual clinics and laboratories serve as primary data collection points. These entities are typically private and operate with their own set of protocols and equipment. Here, ML models are developed and deployed to meet specific laboratory requirements. These models are tailored to address unique challenges and objectives, such as optimizing embryo selection or improving success rates of specific ART procedures.

The local data hubs focus on the following.

3.7.1 Gathering Lab-Specific Data

This includes patient data, procedure outcomes, equipment performance, and environmental conditions within the lab.

3.7.2 Developing Custom ML Models

These models are designed to interpret and utilize local data effectively, providing insights and predictive analytics specific to the clinic's operation.

3.7.3 Ensuring Data Privacy

Local hubs handle sensitive patient data, necessitating stringent privacy and security measures.

3.8 Central Data Collection

Data can be combined across clinics and laboratories in a region that can serve as reference data points. These are typically done in large chains of clinics to derive valuable insights into the entities are typically private and operate with their own set of protocols and equipment. Here, ML models are developed and deployed to meet specific laboratory requirements. These models are tailored to address unique challenges and objectives, such as optimizing embryo selection or improving success rates of specific ART procedures. The central data hubs focus on the following.

3.8.1 Standardizing Data Management and Sharing

It establishes uniform protocols for data sharing and management, akin to the NIH's genomic data sharing policy, ensuring consistency and compatibility across different entities.

3.8.2 Facilitating Data Exchange

The hub enables the sharing of anonymized data, allowing for broader research and analysis while maintaining individual privacy.

3.8.3 Deploying and Refining ML Models

Centralized data allows for the development of more sophisticated and comprehensive ML models that benefit from a wider dataset, potentially leading to more generalized and robust solutions in ART.

A particularly good example of wonderful usage of a central data hub is IVFpredict (http://www.ivfpredict.com/index-1.html). The individualized prediction generated by IVFpredict is based on the work published in the paper by Nelson and Lawlor in *PLOS Medicine*. Based on the data available in the central data hub in UK, between 2003 and 2007, 163,425 IVF cycles were completed in the UK, 23.4% of which resulted in at least one live birth. The researchers used the data collected by the HFEA on 144,018 of these cycles (the other cycles had missing data) to develop a multivariable logistic regression prediction model (a type of statistical model) for the outcome of IVF. According to this model, a decreased chance of at least one live birth was associated with several factors including increasing maternal age, increasing duration of infertility, and the use of the woman's own oocytes. By contrast, a previous IVF live birth and the use of ICSI were associated with increased chances of success. Importantly, compared with an established multivariable prediction model, which was developed before the introduction of ICSI, the researchers' new prediction model predicted the chance of a live birth following IVF with greater accuracy (Nelson and Lawlor 2011).

Powerful predictor models can be developed and implemented in other developing countries like India. As we know, for developing and implementing any systematic process or algorithm, the prerequisite is that the available data is to be digitized. We shall the significance of the ocean of data or the data lake in forthcoming sections.

3.9 Case Study: Centralized Data Utilization in the ArogyaSetu Application During COVID-19

3.9.1 Contextualizing Centralized Data for Pandemic Management

In the realm of reproductive health and medicine, the use of centralized data hubs is not only pivotal for research but also for practical applications in public health crisis management. The ArogyaSetu application, developed in India during the COVID-19 pandemic, serves as an exemplary case of leveraging centralized data for public health benefits (Khan et al. 2022). This section delves into the intricate process of data preprocessing and integration within ArogyaSetu, highlighting the significant role of centralized data in combating a public health emergency.

3.9.2 ArogyaSetu: A Paradigm of Centralized Data Application

ArogyaSetu, developed by the Government of India, functioned as a digital, contact-tracing application. It collected and processed vast amounts of health and movement data from individuals across the country. This process exemplified several key data preprocessing techniques.

3.9.2.1 Context Establishment

The application gathered contextual information, such as location data and health symptoms, which was crucial in tracing COVID-19 spread patterns.

3.9.2.2 Sanity-Checks and Standardization

Data sanity checks ensured reliability, while standardization-maintained data consistency across diverse demographic and geographic inputs.

3.9.2.3 Anonymization and Privacy

A critical aspect was anonymizing personal data to uphold privacy standards, especially relevant in the sensitive area of health data.

3.9.2.4 Normalization and Visualization

Data normalization ensured comparability, while visualizations provided intuitive insights into the spread of the virus, aiding both public understanding and policy decision-making.

3.10 Overcoming Challenges in Data Preprocessing

The application's development faced various challenges inherent to data preprocessing.

3.10.1 Managing Missing Data

In a country as vast and diverse as India, missing data was a significant issue. Sophisticated algorithms were employed to estimate and interpolate missing information.

3.10.2 Data Unit Disparities

The application had to unify data from various units (e.g., metric and imperial systems) for consistent analysis.

3.10.3 Merging Unstructured Data Sources

Integrating data from disparate sources, such as self-reported symptoms, travel history, and contact tracing, was a complex task requiring robust algorithms.

3.10.4 Outlier Management

Identifying and managing outliers was crucial, especially to prevent false alarms or overlook potential hotspots.

3.11 Impact of Centralized Data in ArogyaSetu

The ArogyaSetu application's deployment demonstrates the profound impact of centralized data in a real-world health crisis. By efficiently preprocessing and integrating diverse datasets, the app played a crucial role in contact tracing, predicting hotspots, and informing policy decisions during the pandemic. Figure 3.1 illustrates the ArogyaSetu dashboard, a testament to effective data visualization and centralized data management.

Note for the Reader: The ArogyaSetu case study serves as a beacon for future applications of centralized data hubs in health and medicine in general. Its success underscores the importance of meticulous data preprocessing and the potential of data-driven approaches in public health initiatives. Similar to COVID RT PCR reports, reproductive health-related reports can be collected or uploaded to data

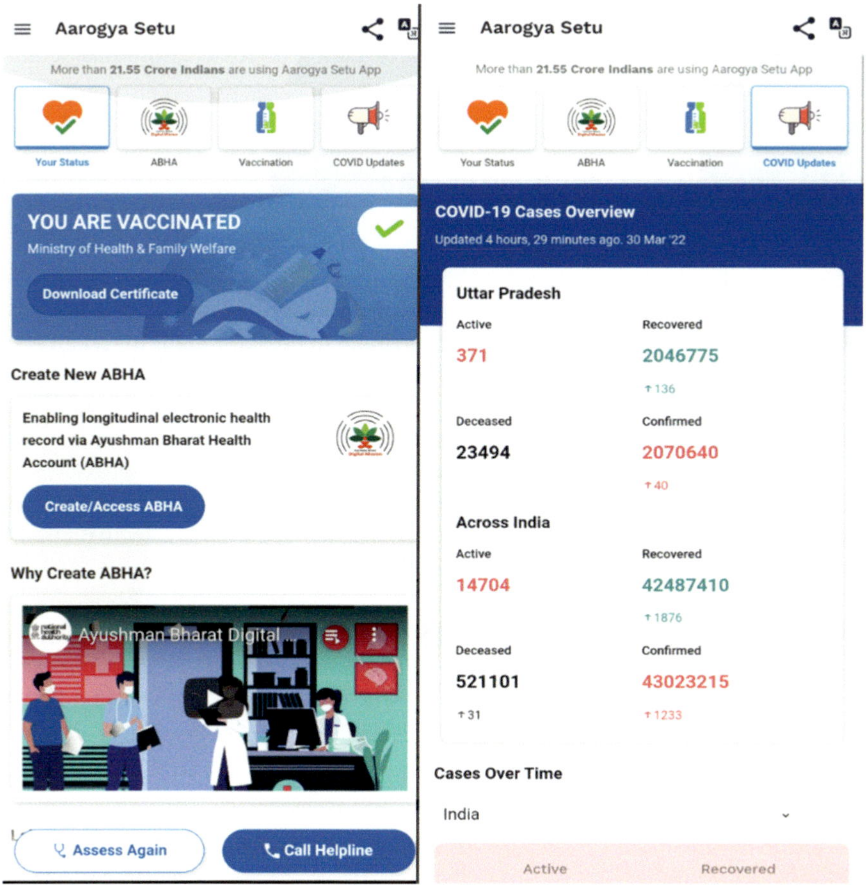

Fig. 3.1 A screenshot of ArogyaSetu mobile application. (Courtesy: ArogyaSetu, Government of India)

hubs from clinics. This data can serve as important steps toward building a tracking system with respect to demographic variations in IVF success rates and respective protocols. Health hazards, e.g., air pollution, nutrition, and good habits correlated to general reproductive health and its demographic variations can be recorded and maintained in a centralized data hub for further processing of big data and getting meaningful insights from the same. Central hub need not be government but can be run by companies that give important indicators to reproductive health-related think tanks that ultimately influence government policy decisions.

3.12 The Tide Is Turning: Why We Need an Ocean of Data in Reproductive Healthcare

Reproductive healthcare is poised for a transformative wave, propelled by the vast and ever-expanding ocean of data. This influx of information promises to revolutionize our understanding of human reproduction, empower patients, and optimize care delivery. However, navigating this sea of data requires careful consideration and ethical responsibility.

3.12.1 The Value of the Ocean of Data

3.12.1.1 Unveiling the Hidden

The sheer volume of data allows us to discover patterns and trends invisible in smaller datasets (Dash et al. 2019). This unlocks secrets of fertility, pregnancy complications, and long-term health outcomes, leading to breakthroughs in research and clinical practice.

3.12.1.2 Charting a Personalized Course

By analyzing individual health records and genetic data, healthcare providers can tailor treatment plans and preventive measures to each patient's unique needs (Earle et al. 2021). This shift towards precision medicine fosters more effective and less invasive interventions.

3.12.1.3 Predicting and Preventing the Storm

Data can be used to predict potential health risks during pregnancy or even before conception (Lee et al. 2016). This empowers proactive interventions that prevent complications and improve outcomes for both mother and child.

3.13 Data in Action: Riding the Waves of Innovation

3.13.1 Electronic Medical Records (EMRs)

Imagine a comprehensive map of a woman's medical history, medications, and allergies, readily available for informed decision-making. EMRs provide this holistic view, empowering patients and healthcare providers alike.

3.13.2 Wearable Devices

These little lifeguards track vital signs, sleep patterns, and activity levels during daily life and also during pregnancy. Real-time monitoring allows for early detection and intervention in potential issues. For example, measuring the heart rate variability (HRV) of a person can be attributed to stress level (Shaffer and Ginsberg 2017). An optimal level of HRV within an organism reflects healthy function and an inherent self-regulatory capacity, adaptability, or resilience. The normal state for a person is when he is not under any stress either physical or mental stress. In a normal state for a person, if the value of HRV is less than 1, then the person is said to be in a stress-free condition where the sympathetic nervous system (SNS) is dominant and if the value of HRV is more than 1, then the person is said to be stressed state at that point of time where the parasympathetic nervous system (PNS) is dominant. Usually, when a person does a lot of physical activity such as exercise, yoga, and more, the body is said to be under a parasympathetic nervous system dominant.

3.13.3 Genetic Testing

This powerful tool can identify patient-specific risks for certain conditions, like chromosomal abnormalities, empowering couples to make informed decisions about family planning and prenatal care.

3.14 Navigating the Ethical Rapids

3.14.1 Privacy and Security

Protecting sensitive health information is paramount. Robust cybersecurity measures and clear data governance frameworks are essential to ensure patient trust and prevent breaches.

3.14.2 Algorithmic Bias

AI algorithms used to analyze data can perpetuate existing biases based on factors like race, socioeconomic status, and geographic location (Char et al. 2018). Mitigating these biases through diverse datasets and transparent algorithms is crucial to ensure equitable access to quality healthcare.

3.14.3 Digital Divide

Unequal access to technology and digital literacy can exacerbate existing disparities in healthcare access (Saeed and Masters 2021). Bridging this gap is essential to ensure everyone benefits from this data-driven revolution.

3.14.4 Conclusion

The ocean of data presents an unparalleled opportunity to transform reproductive healthcare, but navigating its currents requires careful consideration of ethical and practical challenges. By prioritizing patient empowerment, data privacy, and inclusive access, we can harness the power of this information to create a future where everyone benefits from personalized, preventive, and effective reproductive care.

3.15 Data Preprocessing

Data preprocessing plays a critical role in the field of reproductive health, especially in the context of medical big data. It involves various steps such as extraction, cleaning, linking, and storing data from different sources into a single, structured format. This is essential for ensuring the quality and usability of data in large-scale studies, where the characteristics of medical data-like volume, velocity, veracity, and variety-pose significant challenges.

3.15.1 Sanity-Checks, Standardization, Anonymization, and Normalization in Data Preprocessing

3.15.1.1 Sanity-Checks: Ensuring Data Validity

Sanity-checks in data preprocessing are akin to a physician's initial diagnosis before a treatment plan. They ensure that the data being used for reproductive health studies are consistent, credible, and usable. For instance, a common sanity-check in reproductive health data might involve verifying the age range of patients. If a dataset includes ages outside plausible limits (e.g., a patient listed as 120 years old), it signals a need for data cleaning. *Example*: A study on fertility rates might discard data entries where the age of female participants is listed below 12 or above 60, as these are generally outside the typical reproductive age range.

3.15.1.2 Standardization: Harmonizing Data Formats

Standardization in data preprocessing is like speaking a common language in a diverse group. It involves converting data into a consistent format, making it easier to aggregate and compare. In reproductive health, this could mean standardizing units of measurement (e.g., converting all heights from inches to centimeters) or aligning terminology (e.g., using uniform terms for medical conditions). *Example*: An international survey on reproductive health might standardize responses by translating all answers into English and converting all age references to a single format (e.g., years).

3.15.1.3 Anonymization: Protecting Patient Privacy

Anonymization is a critical step in reproductive health data processing, ensuring that individual patient identities are not traceable from the dataset. This involves removing or encrypting personal identifiers such as names, addresses, and social security numbers. *Example*: In a dataset of patients undergoing IVF treatment, anonymization might involve replacing names with unique identifiers and removing specific location details.

3.15.1.4 Normalization: Balancing Data Scales

Normalization in data preprocessing adjusts different scales of data to a common range, enhancing the comparability and effectiveness of machine learning algorithms. In reproductive health, this could involve scaling laboratory values like hormone levels to a standard range, facilitating more accurate cross-sample comparisons. *Example*: When analyzing hormone levels from different labs, normalization helps in adjusting values to a common scale, say 0–1, to accurately compare patient profiles.

This section underscores the pivotal role of these preprocessing techniques in ensuring data reliability and integrity in reproductive health research. By meticulously applying sanity-checks, standardization, anonymization, and normalization, researchers can lay a solid foundation for insightful, data-driven discoveries in reproductive medicine.

3.16 Challenges in Preprocessing Reproductive Health Data

3.16.1 The Intricacies of Handling Missing Data and Data Disparities

In the realm of reproductive health data, the challenge of missing data cannot be overstated. Missing data can arise due to various reasons, such as non-responses in surveys, loss of follow-up in clinical trials, or errors in data collection. This missingness can lead to significant biases in the analysis and interpretation of reproductive health data. One approach to address this issue is through imputation methods, such as multiple imputation or K-nearest neighbors (KNN), where missing values are estimated based on similar data points. For example, in a study examining the impact of lifestyle factors on fertility rates, missing data on exercise frequency could be imputed based on the average exercise frequency of individuals with similar age and BMI. Data unit disparities pose another challenge. Reproductive health data can be sourced from various geographic locations and demographics, often leading to inconsistencies in measurement units and scales. Standardization becomes crucial here. For instance, consider a multi-national study on reproductive age in women, where age is recorded in years in some datasets and in months in others. Converting all data to a standard unit, like years, ensures comparability and consistency in analysis.

3.16.2 Merging Unstructured Data Sources

Integrating unstructured data sources is a critical aspect of data preprocessing in reproductive health. Medical records, patient surveys, and research databases often vary in format and structure. Effective merging of these sources requires robust data transformation techniques to ensure uniformity. For example, integrating text-based patient feedback with structured clinical trial results necessitates natural language processing (NLP) techniques to extract relevant information from the unstructured text and align it with the structured data.

3.16.3 Robust Management of Outliers

Outliers in reproductive health data, whether due to genuine biological variability or measurement errors, can significantly skew results. Identifying and managing these outliers is essential for accurate data analysis. Techniques like Z-score analysis or the Interquartile Range (IQR) method can be employed to detect and handle outliers. For instance, in a dataset analyzing hormone levels across a population, values that deviate significantly from the mean (as determined by Z-scores) could be investigated further to determine if they represent true biological anomalies or data errors.

In conclusion, the preprocessing phase in reproductive health data analysis is fraught with challenges. Addressing these effectively requires a combination of statistical techniques, domain expertise, and a deep understanding of the data's nuances. By overcoming these hurdles, we pave the way for reliable, insightful analyses that can significantly advance the field of reproductive medicine.

Furthermore, the application of data preprocessing in reproductive health is not just limited to enhancing data quality for research but also extends to improving medical data management. For instance, in medical institutions focusing on women and children's health, preprocessing includes activities like ensuring data consistency, integrity, and accuracy across various sources. This is especially crucial when dealing with data from children, who may not have unique identifiers at birth (Dong et al. 2022). Effective preprocessing must include steps to protect the confidentiality of private information, which is of paramount importance in the digital age.

3.17 Data Cleaning and Quality Control in Reproductive Health Datasets

Data cleaning is a fundamental step in the preprocessing phase, especially in the field of reproductive health, where data accuracy is paramount. Handling missing values, outliers, and noisy data efficiently can significantly enhance the quality and reliability of the analyses that follow.

3.17.1 Missing Values

Missing data in reproductive health datasets can arise due to various reasons such as non-responses in surveys, errors in data collection, or loss during data transmission. To address this, one can employ techniques such as the following.

3.17.1.1 Imputation

This involves substituting missing values with estimated ones. For instance, the mean imputation replaces missing values with the mean of the available data. This method, however, may not always be suitable for reproductive health data due to its sensitivity to outliers.

3.17.1.2 Prediction Models

Advanced methods like K-nearest neighbors (KNN) or regression models can predict and fill missing values based on similar data points or established relationships within the dataset.

3.17.2 Outliers

Outliers are data points that significantly differ from other observations. In reproductive health datasets, they might represent rare but important cases, or they could be errors. Techniques for handling outliers include the following.

3.17.2.1 Z-Score Analysis

This method identifies outliers by measuring their standard deviations from the mean. A threshold, typically set at $Z > 3$, flags extreme values.

3.17.2.2 IQR Method

The Interquartile Range (IQR) method uses quartiles to detect outliers. Values that fall below Q1 − 1.5xIQR or above Q3 + 1.5xIQR are considered outliers.

3.17.2.3 Noisy Data

Noisy data refers to irrelevant or meaningless data points that can obscure meaningful patterns. Techniques such as smoothing (using rolling averages, for example) or binning (where data is sorted into discrete bins) can help reduce noise.

3.18 Ensuring Data Accuracy, Consistency, and Integrity

Quality control in reproductive health data processing is crucial to ensure that the data is accurate, consistent, and integral. Some of the key measures include the following.

3.18.1 Data Validation Rules

These rules ensure that the data adheres to predefined criteria. For example, a validation rule might stipulate that the age of patients in a fertility dataset cannot be less than 18 years.

3.18.2 Consistency Checks

This involves verifying that the data across different sources or datasets maintain consistency. For instance, if patient records are collected from multiple clinics, their format and units of measurement should be uniform.

3.18.3 Data Integrity Checks

Integrity checks ensure that the data remains accurate and reliable throughout its lifecycle. This includes measures to prevent unauthorized access or alterations to the data.

3.18.4 Application Example

Consider a dataset from a longitudinal study on reproductive health spanning several years. This dataset might contain instances of missing values (e.g., follow-up information for some participants), outliers (such as rare medical conditions), and noisy data (like incorrectly entered dates). Through careful application of the mentioned data cleaning techniques and quality control measures, researchers can refine this dataset, making it a robust foundation for further analysis, such as identifying trends in reproductive health over time.

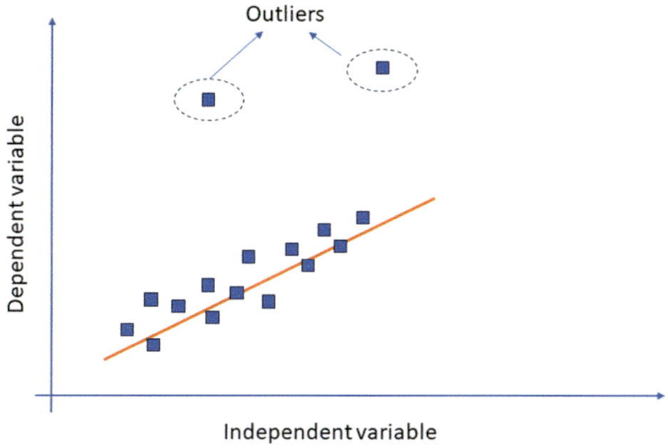

Fig. 3.2 An example of an outlier in data processing

To illustrate, Fig. 3.2 showcases a visual representation of outliers. This graph highlights data points that significantly deviate from the typical range, allowing researchers to scrutinize these cases more closely.

This section provides an overview of essential data cleaning and quality control techniques in the context of reproductive health datasets. The application of these methods ensures the reliability and validity of the data, which is crucial for any subsequent analysis or modeling in the realm of reproductive health and medicine.

3.19 Data Transformation and Feature Engineering

Data transformation is a fundamental step in the preprocessing of reproductive health data, ensuring that this information is suitable for detailed analysis. Key methods include normalization, standardization, and log transformation, each serving a unique purpose in refining data.

Normalization involves scaling individual samples to have a unit norm. This technique is particularly useful in reproductive health data, where measurements can vary widely in scale. For instance, hormone levels measured in different units across various laboratories can be normalized for consistent comparison.

Standardization, on the other hand, involves rescaling data to have a mean of zero and a standard deviation of one. This is crucial when dealing with features that have different scales and ranges. In reproductive health, standardization is vital when integrating patient age, BMI, and hormone levels into a unified analysis framework.

Log transformation is another powerful technique, especially for managing skewed data distributions. It's commonly applied in scenarios where certain reproductive health parameters, such as sperm concentration or follicle counts, exhibit exponential growth or decline. By applying a log transformation, these parameters can be linearized, making patterns more discernible and analysis more robust.

3.20 Introduction to Feature Engineering Techniques

Feature engineering is the process of transforming raw data into features that better represent the underlying problem to predictive models, resulting in improved model accuracy. In reproductive health, this step is crucial for deriving meaningful insights from complex datasets.

One key aspect of feature engineering is featuring creation. For example, combining the age of the patient with their hormonal levels could yield a new feature reflecting reproductive potential. Similarly, interaction terms between lifestyle factors and genetic predispositions can provide deeper insights into fertility-related issues.

Another significant aspect is dimensionality reduction, which simplifies models without losing predictive power. Techniques like Principal Component Analysis (PCA) can be applied to reproductive health data, such as genetic information or high-dimensional imaging data, to extract key features that influence outcomes like pregnancy rates or disease progression.

Additionally, temporal features in reproductive health data, such as menstrual cycle patterns or time-to-pregnancy, can be engineered to capture time-dependent changes. Techniques like time-series analysis can unveil patterns in cycle regularity or identify optimal timing for interventions.

In conclusion, data transformation and feature engineering are pivotal in preparing reproductive health data for analysis. These techniques not only enhance the quality and interpretability of the data but also unlock new dimensions of analysis, crucial for advancing the field of reproductive medicine.

3.21 Dimensionality Reduction in Reproductive Health Data Analysis

In the dynamic field of reproductive health and medicine, the effective analysis of vast and complex datasets is crucial. These datasets, often high-dimensional, can pose significant challenges in terms of computational efficiency and interpretability. This is where dimensionality reduction techniques come into play, serving as a pivotal preprocessing step in data-driven reproductive health research. This section delves into the essence of dimensionality reduction, exploring various methods and their applicability in simplifying reproductive health datasets while retaining essential information.

Dimensionality reduction refers to the process of reducing the number of variables or features in a dataset. In reproductive health, datasets often contain a multitude of variables, from patient demographics to intricate biological markers. High dimensionality can lead to the "curse of dimensionality," which hampers effective data analysis and model performance. Dimensionality reduction helps in mitigating this issue by identifying and retaining the most significant features, thereby simplifying the dataset without substantial loss of information.

3.21.1 Principal Component Analysis (PCA)

PCA is a widely used technique for reducing dataset dimensionality. It works by transforming the original variables into a new set of variables, the principal components, which are uncorrelated and ordered such that the first few retain most of the variation present in the original variables. In the context of reproductive health, PCA can be instrumental in analyzing complex datasets like genomic data, where it can uncover patterns and relationships that are not immediately apparent.

Example: In a study analyzing ovarian reserve markers in fertility research, PCA could be employed to reduce the numerous biomarkers to a smaller set of components, thus simplifying the analysis without overlooking critical information.

3.21.2 t-Distributed Stochastic Neighbor Embedding (t-SNE)

t-SNE is a non-linear dimensionality reduction technique particularly well-suited for the visualization of high-dimensional datasets. It is adept at preserving the local structure of data and revealing hidden patterns in the data. In reproductive medicine, t-SNE can be used to visualize patient subgroups based on complex clinical data, thereby aiding in identifying distinct patterns in patient responses to treatments or in disease progression. *Example*: Consider a dataset with multiple patient characteristics and treatment outcomes. t-SNE could be applied to visually cluster patients into groups based on similarities in their data, thus aiding in the identification of specific subgroups that respond similarly to certain treatments.

3.21.3 Feature Selection Methods

Feature selection involves choosing a subset of relevant features for use in model construction. This method is particularly useful in reproductive health data where some variables might be redundant or irrelevant. Techniques like backward elimination, forward selection, and recursive feature elimination are commonly used. These methods help in improving model interpretability and can also enhance the performance of predictive models. *Example*: In predictive modeling for preterm birth risk, feature selection can be used to identify the most relevant factors from a broad range of clinical and lifestyle-related variables. This not only simplifies the model but also focuses the analysis on the most impactful variables.

3.21.4 Challenges and Considerations

While dimensionality reduction is invaluable, it comes with challenges. The choice of method depends on the dataset characteristics and the research question. Care must be taken to ensure that the reduction process does not oversimplify the data or omit critical information. Additionally, interpreting the results of techniques like PCA and t-SNE requires expertise, as the transformed features may not have a direct or intuitive meaning.

3.21.5 Closure

Dimensionality reduction is a fundamental aspect of preprocessing in reproductive health data analysis. Techniques like PCA, t-SNE, and feature selection methods enable researchers to manage high-dimensional data effectively, facilitating clearer insights and more robust models. However, the application of these methods requires careful consideration to ensure that the essence of the data is preserved and accurately interpreted. With these tools, researchers in the field of reproductive health can continue to advance our understanding and improve patient outcomes through data-driven insights. Overall, the significance of data preprocessing in reproductive health lies in its ability to transform raw, often complex, and unstructured data into a format that is conducive to in-depth analysis and research (Wang et al. 2019). This enables healthcare professionals and researchers to derive meaningful insights, which can lead to improved health outcomes in the field of reproductive health.

3.22 Integration of Reproductive Health Data

The significance of data integration in reproductive health is multifaceted and critical for enhancing service delivery and improving health outcomes. Data integration in this context refers to the process of combining various types of data from different sources into a unified system (Sheahan et al. 2021). This process is particularly important in sexual and reproductive health services, where integration can lead to increased service offers and uptake, potentially improving clinical outcomes. This integration offers a holistic view, essential for effective analysis and decision-making in reproductive medicine.

3.23 Need for Verification During Integration

During data integration, verification is crucial to ensure the accuracy and reliability of the combined dataset. Verification involves several key steps.

3.23.1 Source Authentication

Confirming the legitimacy of data sources to prevent the integration of erroneous or fraudulent data.

3.23.2 Data Consistency Checks

Ensuring that data from different sources is consistent in format, scale, and meaning. For instance, if one source records weight in kilograms and another in pounds, a standard unit must be adopted.

3.23.3 Temporal Alignment

Aligning data points in time, particularly important in reproductive health where timelines (such as menstrual cycles or gestational periods) are crucial.

3.23.4 Ethical Compliance

Ensuring that data integration adheres to ethical guidelines, particularly in handling sensitive patient information.

3.24 Spurious Correlations: A Humorous Take

Ah, spurious correlations—the bane and the comedy of statistical analysis! They're like finding a pattern between the number of times you blink and the stock market fluctuations—intriguing but utterly misleading.

For example, imagine a study that finds a high correlation between the consumption of ice cream and the success rate of IVF treatments. One might be tempted to stock the fertility clinic's freezer with ice cream tubs! But alas, further analysis reveals that the study was conducted during summer when both ice cream consumption and IVF treatments happened to increase. So, unless we believe that ice cream has some magical fertility properties (spoiler: it doesn't), this is a classic case of a spurious correlation.

Or consider the fictional discovery that people who read more romance novels have a higher number of children. Before you rush to add a library to every fertility clinic, it's worth noting that perhaps people with larger families just have more time (or less time, depending on how you view it) for leisure reading.

3.25 Mitigating Risks

To mitigate the risks of spurious correlations, see the following.

3.25.1 Contextual Analysis

Always interpret data within the broader context. Remember, correlation does not imply causation, especially if the correlation is between your morning coffee and global warming trends.

3.25.2 Statistical Rigor

Employing robust statistical methods, including regression analysis and control for confounding variables, can help in distinguishing genuine correlations from those as absurd as correlating your shoe size with your likelihood of winning the lottery.

3.25.3 Expert Review

Involving domain experts in the analysis process is crucial. They can provide insights that are not immediately apparent through statistical analysis alone, such as confirming that chocolate consumption doesn't increase the chances of winning the Nobel Prize (Maurage et al. 2013).

3.25.4 Continuous Monitoring

Regularly reviewing and updating the integrated dataset and analysis methods to incorporate new findings and feedback, and to ensure we're not concluding that wearing socks reduces the risk of catching a cold (unless they're magic socks, of course).

The integration of reproductive health data, when done with meticulous verification and an awareness of the pitfalls of spurious correlations, can lead to profound insights and advancements in the field of reproductive medicine. This integrated approach, underpinned by robust data preprocessing techniques, sets the stage for leveraging bioinformatics and machine learning methods in understanding and enhancing reproductive health outcomes. Overall, data integration in reproductive health is crucial for streamlining services, enhancing research capabilities, and ultimately improving the quality of care and health outcomes for patients. However, achieving effective integration requires overcoming infrastructural, legal, and policy challenges, as well as ensuring the availability of resources and training for healthcare providers.

3.26 The Dashboard: Facilitating User Interaction and Insight Visualization

In the realm of reproductive health data management, the efficacy of data processing and analysis significantly hinges on the accessibility and comprehensibility of the data. This is where the concept of a "Dashboard" comes into play, serving as a vital component in the data hub of "Data-Driven Reproductive Health: Role of Bioinformatics and Machine Learning Methods."

3.26.1 User-Friendly Interface

The dashboard is ingeniously designed to provide a user-friendly interface, allowing users from diverse backgrounds—including clinicians, researchers, and policymakers—to interact seamlessly with the data hub. This interface is not just a gateway to the data but a sophisticated tool that simplifies complex datasets into more understandable formats. For instance, a researcher looking into fertility rates can easily navigate through different data categories, such as demographic information or clinical trial results, without needing extensive technical expertise.

Consider the example of Dr. Deepa Hanamsagar, a reproductive health specialist. When accessing the dashboard, Dr. Deepa Hanamsagar is greeted with a clean, intuitive layout as shown in Fig. 3.3. Key metrics are highlighted upfront, and a simple navigation bar guides her to various datasets. This ease of access is not just a matter of convenience but a crucial factor in ensuring that decisions are made based on the most relevant and current data (Bhargav et al. 2019).

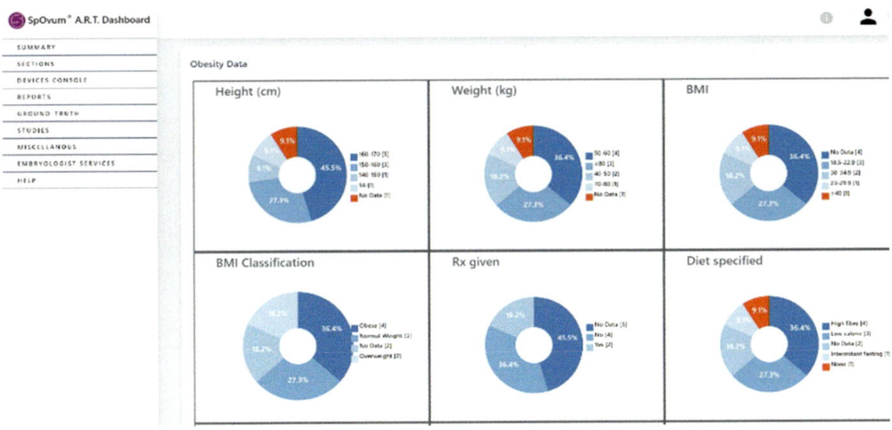

Fig. 3.3 A screenshot of a typical ART dashboard. (Image shared with permission from SpOvum Technologies Private Limited)

3.26.2 Report Generation

Another pivotal feature of the dashboard is its ability to generate comprehensive reports. These reports can be customized according to the user's requirements. For example, a policy-maker looking to understand the impact of a new fertility treatment policy can generate a report comparing pre- and post-policy implementation data. This report can include various parameters such as success rates, demographic impact, and side effects observed, presented clearly and concisely. Visual aids like graphs and charts are integral to these reports, transforming rows of data into visual narratives that are far more digestible. For instance, a line graph showing the trend in fertility rates over the years immediately offers more insight than a table full of numbers.

3.26.3 Visualization of Insights

The true power of the dashboard lies in its capability to visualize insights. Data visualization is not merely an aesthetic aspect; it's a crucial tool for understanding complex patterns and relationships within the data. In reproductive health, where data ranges from patient medical records to large-scale demographic surveys, visualizations aid in uncovering hidden trends and correlations. For instance, a heat map could be used to display regional variations in birth rates, effectively illustrating disparities and trends that might be lost in traditional data tables. Similarly, scatter plots could reveal correlations between various factors affecting reproductive health, such as age, socioeconomic status, and access to healthcare facilities.

These visual tools are not just for data scientists but are designed to be interpretable by all stakeholders in the reproductive health domain. By converting complex datasets into visual formats, the dashboard bridges the gap between data science and practical application, ensuring that insights derived from the data hub are not just accessible but also actionable.

The summary is that the dashboard in the context of reproductive health data management is more than just a user interface. It is the linchpin that connects data with decision-makers, encapsulating the essence of data-driven healthcare. By providing an intuitive interface, robust report generation, and insightful visualizations, it plays a critical role in the effective utilization of data for advancing reproductive health outcomes.

3.27 Harnessing the Power of Data in Assisted Reproductive Technology

As we conclude this chapter on "Preprocessing and Integration of Reproductive Health Data," it is essential to reflect on the transformative potential of machine learning and bioinformatics in the realm of reproductive medicine. The journey from digitizing physical records to the sophisticated management of a data centralization hub underscores the evolution of data handling in assisted reproductive technology (ART).

The transition from traditional paper-based records to digital formats is not just a technological upgrade but a paradigm shift. With machine learning algorithms, we can expedite data entry while enhancing accuracy and reinforcing data integrity. For instance, consider the case of a clinic transitioning to digital records. Here, machine learning models can be trained to recognize and digitize handwritten notes, thus preserving valuable historical data while making it more accessible and analyzable.

The data centralization hub is at the heart of this digital transformation. By harmonizing data from various sources, such as human and device inputs, across the patient journey, it serves as a foundational platform for data management, analysis, and research. This centralization is pivotal for maintaining data integrity and ensures that the information is readily available for various applications. The integration of data from wearable fertility trackers with clinical data is an excellent example of this harmonization, offering a more comprehensive view of a patient's reproductive health.

Data preprocessing techniques within the hub, including context establishment, sanity checks, standardization, anonymization, normalization, and visualization, are critical for quality control. These steps ensure the readiness of data for further analysis and research. The challenge of managing missing data, disparities in data units, merging unstructured data sources, and robust outlier management are central to this phase. An example of this can be seen in the normalization process, where hormone levels measured in different units across various labs are standardized, allowing for meaningful comparisons and analyses.

The dashboard, with its user-friendly interface, exemplifies the application of these complex processes in a practical and accessible manner. It not only facilitates data interaction but also enhances the decision-making process through effective report generation and visualization of insights. For instance, visualizing treatment outcomes across different demographics can provide invaluable insights into the efficacy of various ART protocols.

In the realm of ART, the accurate and efficient handling of reproductive health data is not just a technical necessity but a cornerstone for advancing research, patient care, and operational aspects. These advancements in data handling and analysis have the potential to revolutionize reproductive medicine. The integration of machine learning and bioinformatics in managing and analyzing reproductive health data is not merely an enhancement of existing practices but a necessary step towards a more data-driven and patient-centric approach in ART. Through these innovations, we are not only optimizing the quality and utility of data but also paving the way for personalized medicine in reproductive health. As we harness the power of data, we open new horizons in understanding, diagnosing, and treating fertility issues, ultimately contributing to the well-being of individuals and families. The future of reproductive medicine lies in our ability to effectively integrate and leverage these technological advancements, thereby transforming the landscape of fertility treatments and reproductive health care.

Acknowledgments The authors would like to acknowledge the use of AI-based tools such as Quillbot and Grammarly to improve readability and summarize some parts of the text. The authors have further reviewed the text and take full responsibility for the text.

Conflict of Interest The authors have no conflicts of interest to declare that are relevant to the content of this chapter.

References

Bharadwaj KKS, Rokade SV, Yaswanth GBSV et al (2022) A novel device to micromanipulate oocytes during intracytoplasmic sperm injection. JRHM 3:6. https://doi.org/10.25259/JRHM_4_2022

Bhargav S, Babu RTJ, Chandarkar S et al (2019) A novel technique of using mechanical grippers to immobilize embryo during biopsy. Fertil Steril 112:e291–e292. https://doi.org/10.1016/j.fertnstert.2019.07.855

Bishop CM (2016) Pattern recognition and machine learning, softcover reprint of the original 1st edition 2006 (corrected at 8th printing 2009). Springer, New York

Casella G, Berger RL (2002) Statistical inference, 2nd edn. Thomson Learning, Australia, Pacific Grove

Char DS, Shah NH, Magnus D (2018) Implementing machine learning in health care—addressing ethical challenges. N Engl J Med 378:981–983. https://doi.org/10.1056/NEJMp1714229

Dash S, Shakyawar SK, Sharma M, Kaushik S (2019) Big data in healthcare: management, analysis and future prospects. J Big Data 6:54. https://doi.org/10.1186/s40537-019-0217-0

Dong T, Zhu M, Li R, Wang X (2022) Challenges of utilizing medical big data in reproductive health research. Front Reprod Health 4:800760. https://doi.org/10.3389/frph.2022.800760

Earle S, Marston HR, Hadley R, Banks D (2021) Use of menstruation and fertility app trackers: a scoping review of the evidence. BMJ Sex Reprod Health 47:90–101. https://doi.org/10.1136/bmjsrh-2019-200488

Fox J (2016) Applied regression analysis and generalized linear models, 3rd edn. SAGE Publications, Thousand Oaks

Freedman D (2003) From association to causation: some remarks on the history of statistics. In: Stochastic musings, 1st edn. Psychology Press, p 27

Goodfellow I, Bengio Y, Courville A (2016) Deep learning. The MIT Press, Cambridge, MA

Hastie T, Tibshirani R, Friedman J (2009) The elements of statistical learning. Springer, New York

James G, Witten D, Hastie T, Tibshirani R (eds) (2013) An introduction to statistical learning: with applications in R. Springer, New York

Khan S, Vyawahare C, Singla K, Singh G (2022) The Aarogya Setu mobile application as a bodyguard against COVID-19. J Family Med Prim Care 11:4115. https://doi.org/10.4103/jfmpc.jfmpc_2098_21

LeCun Y, Bengio Y, Hinton G (2015) Deep learning. Nature 521:436–444. https://doi.org/10.1038/nature14539

Lee SH, Nurmatov UB, Nwaru BI et al (2016) Effectiveness of mHealth interventions for maternal, newborn and child health in low– and middle–income countries: systematic review and meta–analysis. J Glob Health 6:010401. https://doi.org/10.7189/jogh.06.010401

Maurage P, Heeren A, Pesenti M (2013) Does chocolate consumption really boost Nobel award chances? The peril of over-interpreting correlations in health studies. J Nutr 143:931–933. https://doi.org/10.3945/jn.113.174813

Nelson SM, Lawlor DA (2011) Predicting live birth, preterm delivery, and low birth weight in infants born from in vitro fertilisation: a prospective study of 144,018 treatment cycles. PLoS Med 8:e1000386. https://doi.org/10.1371/journal.pmed.1000386

Saeed SA, Masters RM (2021) Disparities in health care and the digital divide. Curr Psychiatry Rep 23:61. https://doi.org/10.1007/s11920-021-01274-4

Shaffer F, Ginsberg JP (2017) An overview of heart rate variability metrics and norms. Front Public Health 5:258. https://doi.org/10.3389/fpubh.2017.00258

Sheahan KL, Orgill-Meyer J, Speizer IS et al (2021) Development of integration indexes to determine the extent of family planning and child immunization services integration in health facilities in urban areas of Nigeria. Reprod Health 18:47. https://doi.org/10.1186/s12978-021-01105-y

Till S, Mkhize M, Farao J et al (2023) Digital health technologies for maternal and child health in Africa and other low- and middle-income countries: cross-disciplinary scoping review with stakeholder consultation. J Med Internet Res 25:e42161. https://doi.org/10.2196/42161

Wackerly DD, Mendenhall W, Scheaffer RL (2008) Mathematical statistics with applications, 7th edn. Thomson Brooks/Cole, Belmont

Wang R, Pan W, Jin L et al (2019) Artificial intelligence in reproductive medicine. Reproduction 158:R139–R154. https://doi.org/10.1530/REP-18-0523

Multi-Omics Approaches for Reproductive Health Data

4

Soumya V. Menon, Geeta Joshi, Subash Khadka, Pushkar Joshi, Yashwanth Narayan, Nikhileshwar Krishnan Mahalingam, and Mukund Bhandari

Abstract

The chapter discusses an introduction to different omics techniques and their relevance to their application in reproductive health. Further, the chapter delves into exploring the role of genetics in reproductive problems and investigates the gene expression dynamics in reproductive development and biomarker prediction through proteomics analysis. The chapter also focuses on each of these technologies and their applications individually to the field of reproductive health. The chapter talks about an important aspect of data analysis is the integration of multi-omics data which provides a holistic understanding of reproductive health and its related processes. Furthermore, the chapter also lists important resources for multi-omics data integration and case studies which discuss the successful integration of multi-omics technologies in reproductive health. In the last section, successful applications of multi-omics in clinical settings are discussed. In conclusion, the potential of multi-omics technologies to revolutionize reproductive healthcare is immense and offers exciting prospects for the years ahead.

S. V. Menon · Y. Narayan · N. K. Mahalingam
Department of Chemistry & Biochemistry, School of Sciences, Jain (Deemed-to-be) University, Bangalore, Karnataka, India

G. Joshi
Department of Medical Education, UT Health San Antonio, San Antonio, TX, USA

S. Khadka
Department of Cell System Anatomy, UT Health San Antonio, San Antonio, TX, USA

P. Joshi
Webster University San Antonio, San Antonio, TX, USA

M. Bhandari (✉)
Greehey Children's Cancer Research Institute, UT Health San Antonio, San Antonio, TX, USA
e-mail: bhandarim@livemail.uthscsa.edu

A. Sengupta et al. (eds.), *Data-Driven Reproductive Health*,
https://doi.org/10.1007/978-981-97-7451-7_4

Keywords

Multi-omics · Reproductive health · Bioinformatics · Personalized medicine High-throughput technologies

4.1 Introduction to Multi-Omics in Reproductive Health

4.1.1 Introduction to Multi-Omics

Multi-omics is a term that encompasses multiple "omics" fields within biology, each focusing on the comprehensive study of different types of molecules. Examples of these "omics" fields include genomics, transcriptomics, proteomics, metabolomics, and epigenomics, which respectively examine genes, RNA, proteins, metabolites, and epigenetic marks. "Multi-omics" represents an approach to biological and medical research that integrates data from multiple omics fields simultaneously. This approach aids researchers in gaining a better understanding of complex biological systems by exploring the relationships between various molecular layers (Franchini and Pollard 2017). Multi-omics can unveil new insights into the functioning of living organisms, the development of diseases, and the discovery of novel treatments. It finds applications across various scientific disciplines, such as genomics, cancer research, personalized medicine, and systems biology.

In the context of reproductive health, multi-omics plays a crucial role by providing insights into how different types of molecules interact to influence fertility, pregnancy, and related matters. Below we discuss the use of multi-omics in the study of reproductive health.

4.1.2 Relevance to Reproductive Health

A new approach to biology called "Multi-omics" examines various molecule kinds in a connected manner as shown in Fig. 4.1.

Recent years, from 2020 to 2023, have seen a huge increase in popularity due to advancements in technology, an abundance of data, and a growing understanding of intricate relationship between different biomolecules and molecular pathways. A brief summary of each omics technology and their salient features are summarized in Table 4.1.

By enabling simultaneous analysis of the genome, transcriptome, proteome, metabolome, and epigenome, Multi-omics helps us address this issue and provides a more thorough understanding of biology. Multi-omics is expanding rapidly due in large part to advancements in technology that enable quick and affordable measurement of several types of molecules. For instance, next-generation sequencing (NGS) and other genomic sequencing technologies may generate large amounts of genetic data quickly.

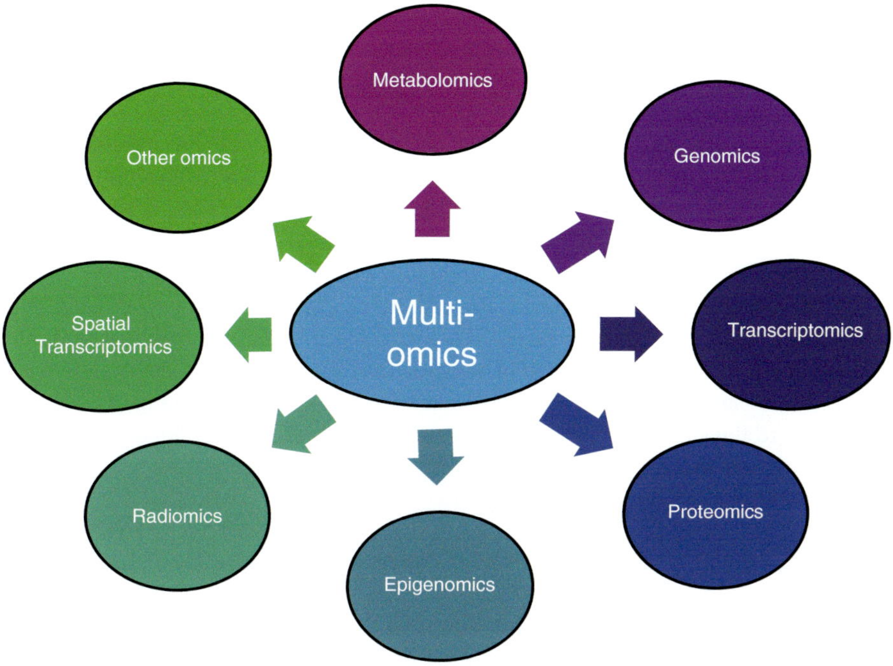

Fig. 4.1 Common omics technologies applied in reproductive health

Table 4.1 Summary of each omics technology and their salient features

Multi-omics type	Data type analyzed	Common modalities	Insights from omics
Transcriptomics	cDNA, RNA	PCR, Micro array, RNA-sequencing	Gene expression, Gene fusion, Immune cell profile, Splice events, RNA modifications
Genomics	DNA	Whole genome sequencing, Whole exome sequencing	Copy number, Mutation profile, Structural rearrangements
Proteomics	Protein	Mass spectrometry	Peptide abundance and modifications
Metabolomics	Metabolites	Mass spectrometry and NMR	Biomolecules and metabolites abundance
Epigenomics	DNA, DNA modifications	PCR, RNA-sequencing, Mass spectrometry, Bisulfite, ChIP, ATAC	DNA modifications, location profile
Spatial transcriptomics	RNA	Spatial transcriptomics platforms (Visium, GeoMx etc.), Imaging mass cytometry, H&E staining	Spatial organization of gene expression within the tissue
Radiomics	Radiographic images	MRI, CT, PET, X-ray, Ultrasound	Tissue type, tissue properties, treatment outcomes

Improved understanding of diseases through multi-omics has also resulted in more individualized and efficient treatment plans. We can identify markers for many diseases and treat them more quickly by integrating data from the proteome, transcriptome, and genome. This is particularly helpful in the case of cancer, as individual tumors vary from one another. Our knowledge of intricate biological processes, such as the development of embryos, the operation of the immune system, and the functioning of the brain, has been increased because of multi-omics. We can gain a greater understanding of biology by examining the interactions between genes, proteins, metabolites, and epigenetic markers.

Multi-omics holds great promise for advancing our understanding of reproductive health. Reproductive processes, like becoming pregnant and giving birth, are extremely intricate and rely on the interactions between several types of molecules. Researchers can gain a comprehensive understanding of these processes, identify potential red flags for the diagnosis and treatment of reproductive health issues, and enhance reproductive healthcare by employing multi-omics techniques.

4.1.3 Overview of Omics Technologies in Reproductive Health

4.1.3.1 Exploring the Role of Genetics in Reproductive Problems

Researchers can learn how genetic variations impact fertility, recurrent miscarriages, and other reproductive disorders by employing multi-omics to examine the genome. Understanding the genetic components can help individuals or couples seek advice, determine the possibility of reproductive problems, and come up with personalized treatments.

4.1.3.2 Investigating Gene Expression Dynamics in Reproductive Development

Through the application of transcriptomics, scientists can investigate the regulation of gene expression in the reproductive tissues at various developmental phases, ranging from gamete production to embryonic attachment. Researchers can learn more about the typical processes of reproduction and the potential reasons for infertility by examining differences in gene expression.

4.1.3.3 Finding Biomarkers Through Proteomic Analysis

Proteomics could identify and quantify proteins associated with reproductive health, potentially serving as markers for diseases such as hypertension, hyperglycemia, or preterm birth. Monitoring protein changes aids in early detection, risk assessment, and development of targeted therapy alternatives.

4.1.3.4 Understanding Metabolic Effects Through Metabolomics

Understanding the role that tiny molecules play in metabolic processes through metabolomics can help us better understand how differences in metabolism impact reproductive health. Determining metabolic markers can be useful in assessing an individual's metabolic state and how it relates to their ability to conceive and carry a child to term.

4.2 Individual Omics Technologies and Their Applications

4.2.1 Genomics in Reproductive Health

The investigation of all genes' structure, function, evolution, mapping, and editing—as well as how these genes interact with one another and the environment—is known as genomics. An organism's whole DNA collection is called its genome. Thus, the body holds an entire copy of every three billion base pairs roughly, or letters, that makeup DNA. Male infertility may have a genetic basis due to chromosomal abnormalities, copy number variations, monogenic, polygenic illnesses, Y chromosome microdeletion azoospermia factor (AZF) deletion, or gene mutation. A quarter of male infertility cases are caused by chromosomal abnormalities and Y chromosome microdeletion azoospermia, indicating their involvement in difficulties related to spermatogenesis. To comprehend the molecular perspective of males with severe oligozoospermia and non-obstructive azoospermia (NOA), a recent study examined the genomes of these individuals. Thirty (10.5%) of the 285 patients (oligozoospermia = 48; NOA = 237) had chromosomal abnormalities, including translocations, inversions, and Klinefelter's syndrome (Chen et al. 2021).

Looking at how genes affect fertility, the risk of reproductive problems, and the chance of having genetic diseases that can affect pregnancy. In female reproductive health management, genetic factors account for the variability in perinatal depression, which is much larger than the 32% heritability of non-perinatal depression. Consequently, genomics analyses demonstrate the potential for identifying biomarkers as an objective measure to aid in diagnosis (such as postpartum depression) (Papadopoulou et al. 2019).

Thus, a better prediction, treatment, and valuation of the risk of genetic abnormality transmission through various techniques which are natural or assisted depends on an overview of the genetic reasons for male and female infertility.

4.2.2 Transcriptomics: Exploring Gene Expression

DNA needs to be read, transcribed, or replicated into RNA during the transcriptional phase. Transcripts are the term for gene readouts, and the transcriptome is the sum of all gene readouts found in a cell. RNA comes in a variety of forms (Zhang et al. 2019b).

The primary form is messenger RNA (mRNA), which is essential to the synthesis of proteins. This process involves the transcription of mRNA from genes, which is subsequently transported to the ribosomes. The amino acid letter sequence in the mRNA is read or translated by the ribosomes, which are then put together to form proteins. Moreover, DNA can be translated into RNA molecules other than those that code for proteins. These transcripts may function to regulate and affect the structure of cells. A study that found overlaps between genes linked to preeclampsia and early pregnancy revealed transcriptomics changes related to preeclampsia. Transcriptome patterns linked to high BMI, vitamin D deficiency, and maternal asthma in females (Rolland et al. 2019).

Even in the germ cell development process, the interaction of many proteins drives human reproductive activities. Studying gene transcription at various stages of germ cell development and maturation is crucial. Therefore, research has looked at the expression of gene transcription in the various reproductive organs and plasma in order to get a clear view of pathophysiological mechanism involved in male infertility (Tarca et al. 2021). Recent studies have demonstrated the decreased expression of testes-specific genes such as ZMYND15 (Zinc finger MYND domain-containing protein 15), PRM1 (pheromone-induced membrane glycoprotein), and TNP1 (Transition Protein 1). Franchini and Pollard (2017) wanted to determine whether the testes-specific genes in seminal plasma can act as biomarkers to predict the occurrence of spermatogenesis in NOA. Additionally, it was revealed that in negative sperm retrieval as opposed to positive sperm retrieval, there was a significant drop in the expression of these genes.

Therefore, it was proposed that these genes' expression would be able to predict whether sperm retrieval will be effective. To ascertain whether gene products from spermatogenic cells could be identified in the Sertoli cell-only testes (SCOT), a different study assessed the transcriptome profile of testicular tissues obtained from males with obstructive azoospermia (OA) and non-obstructive azoospermia (NOA) (Franchini and Pollard 2017).

Now that the genes necessary for healthy spermatogenesis and sperm function have been discovered, a transcriptome analysis can be performed to determine the molecular pathways through which healthy spermatogenesis genes can associate and study their contribution to male infertility and female reproductive health. Accessible transcriptome datasets, and the mechanisms by which these genes contribute to this condition will be investigated in future.

4.2.3 Proteomics: Proteins and Reproductive Processes

A valuable field of study called proteomics can be utilized to get detailed information on proteins that are expressed situations. Additionally, not all encoded genes translate into proteins, particularly in certain clinical conditions, hence this technique is crucial.

The study of proteins based on their location, their structure, physiological functions, and regulation under certain circumstances is known as proteomics. Large, intricate molecules known as proteins are necessary for the creation, process, and control of the body's tissues and organs ("A Brief Guide to Genomics," 2022). Proteomics yields results on protein expression under various situations, making it a valuable tool for comprehending many illnesses. Given that semen is a complicated mixture of secretions from the epididymis and spermatozoa, which originate from the testes. The proteome analysis of the prostate gland and seminal vesicles under various situations will provide insight into the underlying causes of the aforementioned pathology.

Models developed using plasma proteomic data more accurately and early in pregnancy predict spontaneous preterm birth with intact membranes compared to other transcriptome models. More than 10 weeks before clinical presentation, indicators for preeclampsia can be found using urinary proteomics. Two such markers are albumin and fragments of SERPINA1 (serine protease inhibitor 1), which are downregulated in gestational hypertension but increased in women with preeclampsia. Vasculitis and cardiovascular disease are two inflammatory diseases that have also been linked to elevated levels (Sriboonvorakul et al. 2022).

Similarly, in metabolic illnesses like diabetes and obesity, proteomics has been utilized to identify the proteins essential for energy metabolism. Proteomics is a helpful technique in the investigation of infertility, as evidenced by the numerous other investigations that have emphasized the significance of finding differently expressed proteins in the uterus, sperm, and seminal plasma of fertile and infertile men. This means that knowing the function of these proteins and how they could influence the pathogenesis of the disease is made easier by identification and quantification of proteins in various diseases.

4.2.4 Metabolomics: Metabolic Pathways in Reproduction

The evaluation of a set of metabolites in cells, tissue or of an organism is known as metabolomics. Metabolites are the tiny chemicals produced by each reaction and are essential to maintaining cell homeostasis. Metabolite production is individualized and provides a moment in time of a cell's physiological and biological processes. The substrates, intermediaries, and final products of metabolism are known as metabolites. Metabolomics denotes a significant representation of a certain phenotype and a major reflection of gene and protein expression (Zhang et al. 2019a).

Measuring the levels of small molecules (metabolites) in reproductive tissues or fluids, and how they change with fertility, pregnancy, and related issues. In female researchers have highlighted four metabolites that rises during preeclampsia: glutamate, hydroxyhexanoylcarnitine, phenylalanine, and alanine. The postpartum serum metabolomics profile shows elevations in glutathione-disulphide, adenylosuccinate, and ATP were linked to depression and are linked to processes involved in energy production, nucleotide biosynthesis, and oxidative stress. In a short metabolomics analysis, ten compounds showed differential expression in female urine sample (Yu et al. 2021).

Furthermore, it was found that metabolites like isopentenylpyrophosphate, 2-phosphoglyceric acid, and γ glutamyl-Se-methylselenocysteine had a negative correlation with sperm deformity rate, and that acylcarnitine expression was positively correlated with sperm concentration and motility. An additional research revealed the modification and analysis of the metabolic profile of seminal plasma from NOA and the males which are fertile revealed the presence of multiple metabolic pathways, including the citric acid cycle, alanine, aspartate, and glutamate metabolism (Tarca et al. 2021).

Moreover, it can aid in the understanding of the pathophysiology of male infertility and diagnosis of female reproductive disorders since metabolic profiling can be used to uncover changed metabolic pathways. These altered metabolic pathways can then be linked to changes in protein expression and function. Therefore, a vital tool in contemporary reproductive medicine is metabolomics.

4.2.5 Epigenomics: Beyond Genetic Code

Studying how gene activity is controlled by epigenetic marks, such as DNA methylation and histone modifications, and how they affect reproductive health. Epigenetic mechanisms have a profound impact on development throughout pregnancy. The fetal methylation profile incidental from mother plasma resembled that, according to methyl omics, methylome of the placenta and maternal plasma bisulphite sequencing may be used clinically to diagnose fetal trisomy (Zhang et al. 2019a).

Many methylation variations are found in genome which is noncoding region and are connected to the overexpression of lncRNAs (long non-coding RNAs). These RNAs may be involved in the developing preeclampsia which is functional since they expressed improperly in the placenta from preeclamptic pregnancies.

4.2.5.1 What Epigenomics Reveals

The study of epigenomics examines how modifications to the histone tail and the addition or deletion of methyl groups impact reproductive processes. Understanding the molecular elements of reproductive health requires an understanding of the epigenetic regulation of genes linked to development and reproduction.

4.2.6 Other Omics

Though there are numerous other pertinent ways, the omics approaches are the most commonly used. Metabolomics study showed that a number of metals such as, Al, Mn, Co, Pb, Ni, Cd, and Mn in the placenta of preeclampsia. Preeclampsia may occur in relation to a Rb deficiency. Despite preeclampsia's hypertensive genesis, the equivalent Ca, P, and Mg contents in controls and cases suggest that mineralization plays a little role in the condition (Tarca et al. 2021).

Pregnancy and the vaginal and gut microbiomes are closely related. The sequencing-based metagenomics research on the human microbiome has revolutionized the study of the microbiota due to the fact that it can generate a vast library of microbial genomes in big hosts like humans, spanning a range of ecological niches (Fettweis et al. 2019).

Pregnancy-related microbiota research is contemporary and extremely relevant for a variety of disorders. For instance, an imbalance in the vaginal microbiome is linked with an elevated risk of pelvic inflammatory disease, and the diagnosis and management of this condition are complicated by polymicrobial etiology.

By combining data from different omics fields, researchers can get a better picture of the complex systems that control reproductive processes. This can help them find clues for diagnosing and treating fertility and pregnancy-related issues, discover new ways of targeting diseases, and improve our knowledge of reproductive health at the molecular level.

In summary, multi-omics can provide light on the molecular aspects of conception, pregnancy, and the issues that surround them. The present work has illustrated the significance of assessing the male infertility from the perspectives of proteomics, metabolomics, genomes, and transcriptomics while also offering a concise summary of four important omics themes. Identifying putative biological pathways or processes by utilizing publicly available transcriptome data (Zhang et al. 2019b). Male infertility is also demonstrated. The physiology of biological processes such as spermatogenesis, spermiogenesis, spermiation, and energy consumption needs to be preserved for normal reproductive potential.

4.3 Integration of Multi-Omics Data

4.3.1 Challenges in Data Integration

Previously, "omics" data referred to the quantification of numerous biomolecules or molecular events of a given type, for example, genomics for DNA, transcriptomics for RNA, epigenomics for DNA modifications, proteomics for proteins or metabolomics for metabolites. Nowadays, apart from these molecular profiles, multi-omics has been expanded to include other types of high-dimensional data, such as imaging (radiomics), FACS/CyTOF (fluorescence-activated cell sorting/cytometry by time of flight) and large-scale phenotyping (phenomics). The successful integration of such a wide range of heterogeneous datasets presents a cascade of challenges, the major ones are briefly described below.

- **Missing data/values:** A major challenge to multi-omics data integration is missing data (when all biomolecules are not measured in all samples) or missing values (when all measurements are not successful). Limitations in cost, sample availability, instrument sensitivity or other experimental factors can result in missing data/values.
- **Data heterogeneity:** Multi-omics data containing a variety of datasets from different omics layers with completely different data types and distributions require unique data scaling, normalization, and transformation strategies before they can be integrated.
- **Integration with non-omics data:** Clinical/epidemiological data are crucial in characterizing health issues including reproductive diseases, which warrants the joint modeling of omics and non-omics data to enhance the algorithm's ability to accurately classify samples or better predict the outcome. However, many factors including the subjective and highly heterogeneous nature of non-omics data as well as their potential interactions with omics data make the integration process further complicated.

The above challenges arise either during data collection or are inherent to nature of the collected data. However, additional challenges pertaining to data annotation, storage and computational resources may arise during the integrative analysis and community distribution of data (López de Maturana et al. 2019; Tarazona et al. 2021). Specific examples include inefficient computation/storage, diverse signal/noise, inconsistent sample annotation, poor biological interpretation, meta-analysis risks etc. (Tarazona et al. 2021).

4.3.2 Strategies for Effective Integration

Techniques that perform integration of data coming from the same sample type but measured at different omics layer can be broadly organized into early or concatenation-based, middle or transformation-based, and late or model-based integration (Ritchie et al. 2015). Early incorporation performs initial concatenation of features across all measured omics layer followed by analysis of the resulting high-dimensional data; middle integration applies some transformation to each omics data before downstream analysis; and late integration analyzes individual omics data, and then introduces a model or algorithm that combines the outputs of each analysis. More recent attempts to categorize integration approaches expand the above categories into early, mixed, late, intermediate, and hierarchical (Picard et al. 2021). Although these classifications are based on more specific characteristics, they are not mutually exclusive and a given method may be difficult to classify (Flores et al. 2023). Based on availability of data labels, increased magnitude of multi-omics data integration models can be "unsupervised", where inferences are drawn from inputs without prior labels, and "supervised", where known phenotype labels are incorporated to improve accuracy of the analyses. Some of the representative tools that are used in multi-omics data integration are summarized in Table 4.2.

Table 4.2 Representative tools that are used in multi-omics data integration

Multi-omics tool	Features
Galaxy-P	A user-friendly online platform for researchers to analyze multi-omics data using various tools and workflows.
Multi-Omics Factor Analysis (MOFA)	MOFA is a statistical framework for integrating multi-omics data to identify common and unique sources of variation across datasets.
Omics Data Integration (OmicsDI)	OmicsDI offers a platform to integrate multiple omics datasets, facilitating search, analysis, and visualization across diverse omics domains.
XCMS Online	A cloud-based platform for preprocessing, aligning, and statistically analyzing metabolomics data, with support for comprehensive multi-omics integration.
Multi-Omics Visualization Platform (MVP)	MVP enables interactive visualization and exploration of multi-omics data, aiding researchers in identifying patterns and relationships.
OmicsNet	A platform for visualizing and analyzing multi-omics data, covering genomics, transcriptomics, proteomics, and metabolomics, with support for network-based analysis.

The choice of integration approach depends on several factors such as the purpose of integration or the biological question, the types of omics data, and the sample type, all of which can impact the tool or package to use. The predominant objectives of multi-omics data integration can be disease subtype identification, detection of disease associated molecular patterns, identification of diagnostic/prognostic markers, drug response prediction, and understanding the underlying regulatory process of the disease/outcome (Athieniti and Spyrou 2023). The purpose of integration determines the required omics data, the select omics data can then be collected. Selecting an integration strategy after collection of random omics data may limit the ability of the integrative analysis to provide the sought insights. Data for each omics layer needs to be carefully QC-ed and verified that they are coming from same sample type (e.g., diseased vs. adjacent normal tissue). Finally, all data needs to be standardized, to ensure consistency and compatibility in the way they are collected, processed, and stored, and harmonized to ensure their mapping to the same ontologies. Finally, the selection of specific method or technique of integration is determined by the dataset and the task at hand and is not easy to be decided a priori and it is recommended to try out different integration approaches (Chicco et al. 2023) as discussed above.

Effective data integration should also address the challenges discussed above. Prior to integrating diverse biomedical/reproductive health data, one should be aware of each of the potential challenges and have the strategies and instruments ready to tackle such challenges. For example, the issue of missing data/value can be addressed with either utilizing missing value compatible integration methods or by utilizing one of the imputation methods (Flores et al. 2023; Tarazona et al. 2021). Simple imputation approaches such as "mean-imputaion" or "zero-values" are generally developed within the context of a single dataset, newer approaches can leverage information across different omics dataset to facilitate imputation (Flores et al. 2023). For example, TDImpute (Zhou et al. 2020) can utilize DNA methylation data (Epigenome) to impute gene expression data (transcriptome), and more recently, the imputation of DNA methylation data and micro-RNA data from gene expression data and gene expression data from DNA methylation data by training connected neural networks on publicly available TCGA datasets. Similarly, diverse signal/noise across datasets require analysis methods to balance power and experimental design. Integration of omics and non-omics (epidemiological/clinical) technology can be done using unique, controlled or joint modeling and has been reviewed elsewhere (López de Maturana et al. 2019).

4.3.3 Case Studies: Successful Integration Examples

A high proportion of true-multi-omics studies are conducted in cancer settings. Accordingly, ample studies with multi-omics integration are available for ovarian cancer in reproductive health arena. Among gynecological malignancies, ovarian cancer (OC) is a highly heterogeneous disease with the highest mortality rate and poorest prognosis due to lack specific early symptoms. High-grade serous ovarian cancer (HGSOC) is the most frequent and lethal subtype of epithelial ovarian cancers (EOC), which represents about 90% of all OCs (Xiao et al. 2022). Following are some examples of multi-omics approaches in reproductive health settings.

A recent study (Lee et al. 2020) utilized clinically defined (laparoscopic assessments) subsets of HGSOC grouped into (i) R0 [no residual disease after primary debulking surgery (n = 10)], (ii) NACT-ER (n = 10), and (iii) NACT-PR (n = 10) based on excellent response (ER) and poor response (PR) to neoadjuvant chemotherapy (NACT) with the aim of potential biomarker identification. Subsequently, multi-omics (genomics, transcriptomics, phosphor/proteomics) as well as tumor-immune profiling data were obtained from tumor biopsies from primary and metastatic sites. Resulting integrative analysis identified NF1 as a potential OC biomarker, which was significantly lower in R0 group compared to NACT group HGSOC samples. Additionally, R0 group was characterized by increased number of infiltrated T-cells and decreased macrophages.

Another study (Zeng et al. 2021) used histopathological images to predict molecular features using CellProfiler and utilized those to establish prediction models by machine learning (ML) methods in training set from TCGA data, and tested the performance of the model in test and validation datasets from TCGA and tissue microarray data to predict overall survival (OS) in HGSOC. The prognostic model based on histopathological image features was able to predict 5-year OS in test set and validation set with area under curve (AUC) more than 70% (AUC >0.7). Combining two omics data (radiomics and genomics) increased the efficiency of the model (AUC = 0.834) while integrating the multi-omics (radiomics, genomics, transcriptomics, and proteomics) data further enhanced the model's efficiency (AUC = 0.911) highlighting the importance of multi-omics integration for more comprehensive and accurate disease insights.

Finally, with the aim of identifying maternal biological modalities associated with preterm birth (PTB, defined as delivery of a live infant before 37 weeks of gestation), this study (Jehan et al. 2020) utilized cell-free transcriptomics, urine metabolomics and plasma proteomics from 81 pregnant women in five different cohorts from low- and middle-income countries (LMICs). They applied a cohort-adjusted ML algorithm to each dataset followed by a higher-level ML model for integrative analysis, which again proved to be more accurate (AUC = 0.83) compared with models derived from independent modalities (transcriptomics: AUC = 0.73, metabolomics: AUC = 0.59, and proteomics: AUC = 0.75). Main features associated with PTB in this study were glutamine/glutamate metabolism and valine/leucine/isoleucine biosynthesis related to metabolic module measured in urine collected early in pregnancy as well as an inflammatory module including IL-6 expression among other cytokines.

4.4 Multi-Omics and Clinical Applications

4.4.1 Infertility and Omics Technologies

Infertility is a problem affecting one in six couples, which is approximately 15% of the population wishing to start a family. In 30% of infertile couples, the male factor is a major cause. Based on the combined approaches of different "omics" mainly functional genomics, proteomics, biochemistry etc. Single-cell omics mainly reflect on profiling of single cell whereas multi-omics allows a systematic understanding and compilation of different omics technologies and can provide an overall view of the pathophysiology of a disease, which has significance for research in the numerous thrust areas of life sciences. However, current multi-omics studies mainly concentrate on the integration and interpretation of various types and sources of data, which are divided into vertical and horizontal aspects according to the type of data integrated. We will be focusing on the integration of omics in the identification and some case study presentations will be highlighted.

Numerous omics technologies have been investigated to identify diagnostic markers but are not yet clinically approved. For example, Zhang et al. (2019b) based on their experiments concluded that the plasma concentration of ADAM12 (A Disintegrin and Metalloproteinase-12) has been found to be changed in several pregnancy-related disorders, but application of ADAM-12 as a marker for adverse outcomes is yet to be clear. Glucocorticoid receptor co-chaperone gene sensitivity in peripheral blood gene expression diminished with the progression of pregnancy and increasing maternal depressive symptoms and may serve as a biomarker for risk of developing depressive symptoms during pregnancy. In genomic studies, genome-wide association studies (GWAS) are aimed to identify the genotypes and phenotypes associated with any particular disease or trait. For example, a GWAS study of 281,416 individuals without diabetes identified 242 loci associated with glycemic traits (Curry et al. 2019). There are a few leading studies on the genetics of PCOS (Fettweis et al. 2019; Kharb and Joshi 2023; Menon and Golgeri 2021). Urinary proteomics can identify biomarkers for preeclampsia more than 10 weeks before clinical presentation. Two such markers are fragments of SERPINA1 and albumin, upregulated in women with preeclampsia but downregulated in gestational hypertension.

Different predictive models are developed for the diagnosis of diseases and syndromes such as PCOS, uterine fibroids etc. Recently, genomics associated/based on the machine learning approach comprises these predictive models for female health complications. Machine learning from transcriptomics and proteomics profiling of plasma and metabolomic analysis of urine allowed accurate predictions of preterm birth and also premature ovarian insufficiency (POI) (Kharb and Joshi 2023).

The disease complexity is a huge challenge when giving the treatment to the males with infertility. From past some decades, role of miRNA in the development and disease has gained attention due to the novel therapeutic approach. MiRNA mainly inhibits the expression of target genes by binding to target mRNA, promoting its degradation or hindering its translation. It is worth mentioning that the target genes of miR-182-5p, such as PRKACB, RGS17, BNC2, and SNX30, have regulatory roles in reproductive system signaling pathways (Jin et al. 2023).

Protein interacting with C-1 Kinase (P1CK1) deficiency in men lead to the damage of acrosome maturation and the multi-omics analysis of P1CK1 knockout mouse model were performed by Jin et al. (2023). They found that this approach could identify some candidate biomarkers for P1CK1 deficient male infertility. Another approach in investigation of infertility is proteomic-based approach as it is the best tool for predictive and comparative analysis of certain specific proteins.

Some of the researchers such as Amaral et al. (2014), Baker et al. (2013), and du Plessis et al. (2011) based on their findings proved that some proteins are involved in the reduction of oxidative stress in males and these proteins can be used as biomarkers in the quality assessment of semen.

4.4.2 Prenatal Development Insights from Multi-Omics

Preterm birth is a syndrome with multiple etiologies and is very complex and difficult to predict by a single set of biomarkers. The most powerful predictor of spontaneous preterm birth is a sonographic short cervix in the mid trimester and a history of spontaneous preterm birth in a prior pregnancy (Romero et al. 2013). The identification of prenatal development and complications are not specifically diagnosed only based on clinical technologies. Hence numerous researchers have opted for the multi-omics approach to treat preterm birth and other obstetrical complications. In view of this, Tarca et al. (2021) made a blood omics-based approach, i.e., transcriptomic model and plasma proteomic profile were generated from 216 women with normal and abnormal pregnancies. Based on the multi-omics platform combined with prediction using sPTD and PPROM they could study the reason for preterm birth and related complications.

Recently, one of the case studies emphasized the application of one of the technologies named array-CGH to screen embryos from both reciprocal and robertsonian translocation carriers for unbalanced translocation derivatives, as well as aneuploidy status of all 24 chromosomes. The study was conducted in 12 different couples having 28 preimplantation genetic diagnosis (PGD) cycles, which resulted in chromosomally balanced pregnancies. Biopsied cells from the day 3 embryos were lysed and the DNA amplified by WGA. WGA products were then processed by array-CGH. Euploid embryos were then selected for transfer on day 5 of the same cycle. The proteomic and metabolomic analysis was performed for the selection of viable embryo, selection of potential embryo and transplant it successfully. Omics technologies are beneficial in exploring the difference among follicles, human gametes, and embryos.

4.4.3 Understanding Gynecological Diseases

Nearly all women experience gynecological problems at some point in their life. It may hurt, and many avoid it as normal pain because it may happen at any time during the menstrual cycle. Due to the pelvic location of the pain, it can also be mistakenly identified as other ailments such as gastrointestinal, musculoskeletal, urinary (interstitial cystitis), or psychogenic (psychological or sexual abuse). The discipline of "integrative genetics" emerged as a result of the development of genotyping arrays, which made it possible to conduct extensive genome-wide association studies and techniques for analyzing global transcript levels. Nowadays, many biological researchers include other omics technologies, such proteomics and metabolomics, into their routine research procedures. When opposed to single omics investigations, multi-omics provides a means of comprehending the information flow underlying disease.

- **Adnexal tumors**: Adnexal tumors are the eighth most frequent cause of cancer-related death in women globally, with over 310,000 new cases and around 200,000 fatalities expected in 2020 (Sung et al. 2021). Growths close to the uterus are called adnexal masses or adnexal tumors. These growths can originate in the connective tissues, fallopian tubes, and ovaries (Menon et al. 2021). Adnexal tumors come in a variety of forms and are classified as benign or malignant based on their location (ovarian or non-ovarian) and level of cancer. Over the last 10 years, a great deal of work has been done by researchers to obtain detailed molecular profiling of adnexal tumors, which can assist direct more accurate and customized therapeutic recommendations. In recent times, advancements in multi-omics technologies such as proteomics, metabolomics, transcriptomics, and genomes have made it feasible to identify and perhaps generate more useful biomarkers for application in the clinical practice. Our understanding of the condition has grown as a result of the integration of multi-omics data, which has also revealed important tumor biomarkers (Li et al. 2020). This emphasized prospective uses of multi-omics for finding novel biomarkers and enhancing clinical assessments, as well as recent developments and viewpoints in the use of multi-omics technology in tumor research.
- **Cervical dysplasia:** A sexually transmitted virus known as the human papillomavirus (HPV) can induce abnormal changes to healthy cells in the cervix, leading to the vagina. This condition is known as cervical dysplasia. These aberrant cells frequently do not have cancer, but if they are not found and treated quickly may become dangerous. The HPV vaccine lowers the chance of developing cervical dysplasia. When cervical dysplasia is discovered, symptoms are uncommon, however irregular bleeding might occasionally happen.

Applying high-throughput approaches to biological samples for differential expression analysis enables the determination of both the physiological state of normal cells and the alterations brought about by the infection of HPV. The term "molecular signature" refers to the cluster of differential molecular profiles in the proteome, transcriptome, or genome that are evaluated in the disease (Zhang et al. 2020). Proteomic analysis of biological samples from individuals with varying degrees of cervical intraepithelial neoplasia (CIN) has helped to uncover cervical proteins linked to cervical dysplasia and clarify the pathways involved in the initiation and progression of diseases.

- **Incompetent cervix endometriosis:** If the cervix dilates early during the first trimester of pregnancy without any pain or contractions, it is known as an incompetent cervix (Chen et al. 2020). While a hereditary weakening of the cervix can be a cause, it is not always the case. Exposure to diethylstilbestrol (DES), an underlying connective tissue disorder, a history of second trimester pregnancy terminations, or a history of cervical procedures (such as loop electrical excision procedure or cone biopsy) can increase the risk of developing an incompetent cervix (Wang et al. 2016). One of the symptoms of this condition can be pelvic pain. In the second and third trimesters of pregnancy, cervical insufficiency (CI) can result in recurrent spontaneous abortion (RSA) and preterm birth (PTB). It is an obstetric syndrome marked by painless, increasing dilatation and cervix shortening.

Using a multi-omics approach, the study investigated alterations in proteins and metabolites in the cervical secretions of individuals with CI for the first time (Chen et al. 2020). The work enhanced the prognosis of CI patients during pregnancy by illuminating the potential pathophysiology of the condition and offering a therapeutic target for early intervention and prevention.

- **Endometriosis:** The endometrium, or tissue that should line the uterus, grows outside of the uterus, resulting in endometriosis. The majority of common growths are found in the bladder, bowels, ovaries, and behind the uterus. Infertility, heavy periods, and pain in the abdomen, lower back, or pelvis are all symptoms of endometriosis. In order to identify susceptible people more accurately in the early stages of the disease, scientists have identified novel biomarkers. In the first instance, the development of genotyping arrays paved the way for extensive genome-wide association studies (GWAS) and the evaluation of global transcript levels, which in turn gave rise to integrative genetics (Han et al. 2020). High-throughput technologies have significantly transformed medical research. Within this paradigm, extensive research has been carried out using the "omics" platforms at various biological levels, enabling a more in-depth molecular resolution reexamination of endometriosis. Omics technologies are capable of detecting and analyzing hundreds of markers in a single experiment. Proteomics and metabolomics have recently been incorporated into the routine methodology of researchers working with gynecologists. More significantly, compared to studies of any single-omics type, multi-omics approach is advantageous to gain insight of the entire information that underlies endometriosis.

4.5 Personalized Medicine in Reproductive Health

4.5.1 The Role of Multi-Omics in Personalized Healthcare

The eras of medicine are constantly evolving and currently we are at the brink of paradigm shift towards precision medicine. Medical practice in the past evaluated signs and symptoms and was based on physician's knowledge (intuition medicine), which is evolving through present day clinical trials (evidence-based medicine) to the future, where algorithms based on patient's clinical and multi-omics data tailor the treatment for each individual patient (precision/personalized medicine) (Pammi et al. 2023).

The stage of paradigm shift is made possible by the rise of multi-omics technologies and sophisticated bioinformatics tools aided by machine learning (ML) and artificial intelligence (AI). Since cracking the genetic codes of human genome through the "Human Genome Project" in 2003, scientists and clinicians started to identify the genetic alterations in human diseases, which also paved the way for DNA and RNA sequencing with high speed and precision but at a low cost. Alongside genomics, use of other omics approaches such as transcriptomics and proteomics allowed the identification of abnormalities at RNA transcription and protein synthesis levels providing a comprehensive understanding of the disease pathogenesis. Multi-omics are available at a resolution of a single cell, which makes them applicable for rare diseases and limiting specimens despite the low sample counts and smaller sample sizes.

Today, scientists can integrate a patient's clinical profile with multi-omics data and other test results by using ML approaches that can link the data from one patient to those from a large cohort of patients. This cross-comparison allows them to predict the disease progression and identify a drug candidate that best treats the specific (subtype of) disease. The accuracy of prediction, however, is dependent on training datasets, the higher the volume and diversity of training data, the more accurate the computational model. So, the predictive algorithms/models based on patient's multi-omics and clinical profile are yet to replace the clinical decision making but are complimenting the clinicians in decision-making. Since multi-omics is what allows the deep characterization of patients and disease states to make targeted treatment possible, it is central to personalized healthcare.

4.5.2 Developing Personalized Treatment Approaches

Precision medicine is not a new concept in reproductive health. The end goal of reproductive medicine is to offer healthy offspring to fertility impaired couples, which has been in practice for decades with assisted reproductive technologies (ART) such as in-vitro fertilization (IVF). In reproductive health arena, precision medicine refers to collection of health history, family history and information on lifestyle and genotype to customize individual treatment protocols, and such a personalized health model enhances the efficiency of assisted reproductive technologies (ART) in place of applying same procedures for treating all patients (Zhang and Yu 2020). Since the first IVF baby, Louise Brown, was born in 1978, many improvements such as embryo cryopreservation, blastocyst stage transfer, single embryo transfer, preimplantation genetic screening (PGS), minimal simulation protocols have been made (Zhang and Yu 2020), each of which are a step towards precision medicine. With the advent of multi-omics and computational tools to integrate the omics data to clinical profile, personalized treatment approaches in reproductive health are becoming more popular.

The relative ease of sample (blood, urine, other fluids, and biopsies) collection in reproductive diseases makes the gathering of multi-omics data more feasible and warrants for the approaches to implement these data towards personalized treatment. As an example, Liang et al. (2016) leveraged the DNA mutation, mRNA- and protein-expression data from a hypermutated hepatocellular carcinoma patient to propose a strategy to identify the driver genes of the disease in that patient. The approach aimed at assessing the impact of tumor mutated allele in the encoded protein function, and based on their set criteria, identified five driver genes in that patient. They further validated their observations with knockout experiments involving those driver genes. Similar approaches can be applied for developing personalized treatment strategies by leveraging the multi-omics data and the power of ML algorithms-based predictive models.

4.5.3 Predictive Modeling for Preventive Medicine

One of the major goals of multi-omics integration is prediction of biomarkers, which are the molecular footprints of the cellular functions in a particular state. Such biomolecules are an integral part of biological pathways that mediate the information flow, and hence can reveal the underlying biology. Integrated multi-omics analysis is an excellent opportunity to identify reliable biomarkers by utilizing information from multiple molecular events.

Given the high dimensionality of omics data, ML methods are needed to extract any insights from these data. ML methods can be unsupervised and supervised, the former tracks patterns in the data while the latter are mainly predictive and explanatory. Supervised methods derive a series of mathematical models from the training dataset, which can then be used to predict the class labels of the distinct validation dataset. In brief, using ML methods for prediction of clinical phenotypes involve collection of training data (clinical, multi-omics) to select the subset of features associated with phenotype of interest, building a multivariate model based on these features, acquiring validation dataset with same omics profiling methods and using them as a new input to the established multivariate model, and finally, using the predictions provided by the model to assess the classification performance of the test input by comparing the model output and the actual clinical phenotypes of the patients in the validation set (Tebani et al. 2016). The biomarkers identified by such supervised ML approaches can be utilized not only in precision treatment but also for the early diagnosis and warranted preventive efforts.

Recently, Li et al. (2022) developed a digital phenotyping algorithm to curate >100,000 pregnancies from electronic medical records (EMR) across a large health care setting and applied ML approaches to a training dataset to construct predictive models of preeclampsia (PE) across pre-, intra-, and postpartum periods. They employed gradient-boosted tree models, which can inherently address the missing values that are ubiquitous in the EMR. Their model was able to successfully predict the PE with high accuracy in two independent validation cohorts across all three pregnancy periods with area under receiver operating curve (AUC) of 0.92, 0.82, and 0.89 at 37 gestational weeks, intra- and postpartum respectively. The ML approach employed identified both known (blood pressure, weight, maternal age) and potentially novel risk factors for PE indicating that the model is not only applicable in earlier identification of PE risk but also sets a good model for promoting precision therapeutic strategies given its higher prediction accuracy than what exists in clinical practice. Moreover, certain "omics" data are reported to be promising in PE identification but these data, although are not routinely collected in the clinic, can certainly be acquired, and then incorporated into such ML models in addition to other inputs such as biomarkers to further enhance the performance accuracy.

4.6 Future Directions and Emerging Trends

4.6.1 Innovations on the Horizon

The current era of multi-omics is the outcome of revolutionary technological advancements of the recent past that enables us to identify numerous biomolecules. The major "omics" like genomics, transcriptomics, proteomics, and metabolomics have generated respective epiomics (epigenomics, epitranscriptomics, and epiproteomics) and interactomics which are technology-based, and other omics such as "immunomics" and "microbiomics" that are knowledge-based. The developmental trend of omics technologies incorporates three facets—ameliorating the technical issues in existing omics (e.g., reducing sample size/amount, enhancing accuracy and reproducibility), deriving novel omics types (e.g., novel epiomics derived from modifications by various intermediate metabolites), and novel knowledge-based omics (e.g., "redoxomics" given the critical role of redox homeostasis in health and disease) (Dai and Shen 2022).

Ever expanding technological innovation has brought the application of multi-omics close to clinical practice. Today, multi-omics is not only applicable to bulk samples but also to dissociated single cells (single cell multi-omics) and is gradually moving towards spatial multi-omics that preserves the spatial information of different cells in an intact tissue. Single cell multi-omics enables discovery of novel cell types, reveals tissue/tumor heterogeneity, and provides the basis for spatial multi-omics, which are crucial to expedite biomarker discovery and gaining disease insights beyond what bulk multi-omics can do. Spatial transcriptomics platforms provided by 10× Genomics can be used for constructing high-resolution microscopic images with transcriptomic data aligned to the tissue footprint and extended for interpreting spatial multi-omics. The reduced cost with enhanced speed and throughput of next-generation sequencing (e.g., Illumina NovaSeq X) alone is a big leap towards making the multi-omics integrated into clinical practice. Along these lines, long-read sequencing technologies, which are available today, can advance the detection of genetic variation in cells. Finally, what is discussed in this section is just a snippet of the current innovations but may serve as indicators of what may be possible soon.

4.6.2 Integrating Machine Learning and AI

Obtaining maximum insights from multi-omics data is limited by the complexity and heterogeneity of such data, which makes integrating them to each other and to clinical and epidemiological data very challenging. This is where ML/AI (artificial intelligence) come into play. The integration of AI/ML has seen significant strides in medicine in the last decades where radiomics taking the top place (Joshi et al. 2024). Using multi-omics ("immunomics" and "microbiomics" included)-based systems biology network analysis and integrating the information with epidemiological patient profile, and clinically disease phenotypes with the use of AI and ML algorithms enables identification of biomarkers to guide personalized interventional strategies for high-risk patients.

Therefore, advanced bioinformatic tools that can handle patient's multi-omics data, methods to integrate patient's non-omics data to multi-omics data, "learn" the patterns from big population data and generate models, and inputting the relevant features from patient data into such model to predict outcomes are central to precision medicine. AI/ML algorithms are the only methods to successfully handle the latter three steps in the process. Therefore, integrating AI/ML in multi-omics analysis is essential.

4.6.3 Future Challenges and Opportunities

Integration of multi-omics data and clinical metadata is set for paradigm shift in comprehensive knowledge of biological processes and the ways medicine is practiced but this comes with its share of challenges. Currently, the major challenges in multi-omics integration are the underlying heterogeneity in individual omics data, cumbersome preprocessing steps with lack of universal standards, large size of data requiring compute intensive tools and big storage space, and lack of robust methods to integrate omics and non-omics data. These challenges are gradually being addressed with the advent of better bioinformatics tools, use of AI/ML in integration approaches, and advanced data storage and sharing platforms. On the other hand, single-cell and spatial multi-omics are in their growth phase and has many challenges such as high cost, low throughput, and limited capture area for spatial technologies are to be addressed in the future. Finally, a review article notes the potential societal and ethical issues related to use of AI in healthcare in the future (Vellido 2019). The author points out issues such as legislation, ethics and fairness, interpretability and explainability and privacy and anonymity, but also warns on other issues such as robustness and safety, economics and accessibility, or complex data management.

These challenges also bring opportunities to develop solutions to address them. Further developments in multi-omics as well as non-omics integration analysis must aim to ease interoperability of multiple datasets and to develop a framework or tools for seamless analysis of heterogeneous data. The societal issues of integrating AI in healthcare calls for the collaboration between the AI/ML and medicine/

healthcare communities in search for the methods, protocols, guidelines, and data analysis pipelines that explicitly take into consideration all these societal issues (Vellido 2019).

Acknowledgments The authors would like to acknowledge the use of AI-based tools such as Quillbot and Grammarly to improve readability and summarize some parts of the text. The authors have further reviewed the text and take full responsibility for the text.

References

(2022) A brief guide to genomics. https://www.genome.gov/about-genomics/fact-sheets/A-Brief-Guide-to-Genomics

Amaral A, Castillo J, Ramalho-Santos J, Oliva R (2014) The combined human sperm proteome: cellular pathways and implications for basic and clinical science. Hum Reprod Update 20:40–62. https://doi.org/10.1093/humupd/dmt046

Athieniti E, Spyrou GM (2023) A guide to multi-omics data collection and integration for translational medicine. Comput Struct Biotechnol J 21:134–149. https://doi.org/10.1016/j.csbj.2022.11.050

Baker MA, Naumovski N, Hetherington L et al (2013) Head and flagella subcompartmental proteomic analysis of human spermatozoa. Proteomics 13:61–74. https://doi.org/10.1002/pmic.201200350

Chen C, Chen C, Sun F (2020) Assessment of the cervix in pregnant women with a history of cervical insufficiency during the first trimester using elastography. Acta Obstet Gynecol Scand 99:1497–1503. https://doi.org/10.1111/aogs.13942

Chen J, Spracklen CN, Marenne G et al (2021) The trans-ancestral genomic architecture of glycemic traits. Nat Genet 53:840–860. https://doi.org/10.1038/s41588-021-00852-9

Chicco D, Cumbo F, Angione C (2023) Ten quick tips for avoiding pitfalls in multi-omics data integration analyses. PLoS Comput Biol 19:e1011224. https://doi.org/10.1371/journal.pcbi.1011224

Curry A, Williams T, Penny ML (2019) Pelvic inflammatory disease: diagnosis, management, and prevention. Am Fam Physician 100:357–364

Dai X, Shen L (2022) Advances and trends in omics technology development. Front Med 9:911861. https://doi.org/10.3389/fmed.2022.911861

Du Plessis SS, Kashou AH, Benjamin DJ et al (2011) Proteomics: a subcellular look at spermatozoa. Reprod Biol Endocrinol 9:36. https://doi.org/10.1186/1477-7827-9-36

Fettweis JM, Serrano MG, Brooks JP et al (2019) The vaginal microbiome and preterm birth. Nat Med 25:1012–1021. https://doi.org/10.1038/s41591-019-0450-2

Flores JE, Claborne DM, Weller ZD et al (2023) Missing data in multi-omics integration: recent advances through artificial intelligence. Front Artif Intell 6:1098308. https://doi.org/10.3389/frai.2023.1098308

Franchini LF, Pollard KS (2017) Human evolution: the non-coding revolution. BMC Biol 15:89. https://doi.org/10.1186/s12915-017-0428-9

Han Y, Li M, Ma H, Yang H (2020) Cervical insufficiency: a noteworthy disease with controversies. J Perinat Med 48:648–655. https://doi.org/10.1515/jpm-2020-0255

Jehan F, Sazawal S, Baqui AH et al (2020) Multiomics characterization of preterm birth in low- and middle-income countries. JAMA Netw Open 3:e2029655. https://doi.org/10.1001/jamanetworkopen.2020.29655

Jin J, Li K, Du Y et al (2023) Multi-omics study identifies that PICK1 deficiency causes male infertility by inhibiting vesicle trafficking in Sertoli cells. Reprod Biol Endocrinol 21:114. https://doi.org/10.1186/s12958-023-01163-w

Joshi G, Jain A, Araveeti SR et al (2024) FDA-approved artificial intelligence and machine learning (AI/ML)-enabled medical devices: an updated landscape. Electronics 13:498. https://doi.org/10.3390/electronics13030498

Kharb S, Joshi A (2023) Multi-omics and machine learning for the prevention and management of female reproductive health. Front Endocrinol 14:1081667. https://doi.org/10.3389/fendo.2023.1081667

Lee S, Zhao L, Rojas C et al (2020) Molecular analysis of clinically defined subsets of high-grade serous ovarian cancer. Cell Rep 31:107502. https://doi.org/10.1016/j.celrep.2020.03.066

Li C, Sun Y-D, Yu G-Y et al (2020) Integrated omics of metastatic colorectal cancer. Cancer Cell 38:734–747.e9. https://doi.org/10.1016/j.ccell.2020.08.002

Li S, Wang Z, Vieira LA et al (2022) Improving preeclampsia risk prediction by modeling pregnancy trajectories from routinely collected electronic medical record data. npj Digit Med 5:68. https://doi.org/10.1038/s41746-022-00612-x

Liang L, Song L, Yang Y et al (2016) Validation of a multi-omics strategy for prioritizing personalized candidate driver genes. Oncotarget 7:38440–38450. https://doi.org/10.18632/oncotarget.9540

López De Maturana E, Alonso L, Alarcón P et al (2019) Challenges in the integration of omics and non-omics data. Genes 10:238. https://doi.org/10.3390/genes10030238

Menon S, Golgeri B (2021) A review on polycystic ovarian syndrome in relation to insulin resistance. Pathogenesis:24–31

Menon U, Gentry-Maharaj A, Burnell M et al (2021) Ovarian cancer population screening and mortality after long-term follow-up in the UK Collaborative Trial of Ovarian Cancer Screening (UKCTOCS): a randomised controlled trial. Lancet 397:2182–2193. https://doi.org/10.1016/S0140-6736(21)00731-5

Pammi M, Aghaeepour N, Neu J (2023) Multiomics, artificial intelligence, and precision medicine in perinatology. Pediatr Res 93:308–315. https://doi.org/10.1038/s41390-022-02181-x

Papadopoulou Z, Vlaikou A-M, Theodoridou D et al (2019) Unraveling the serum metabolomic profile of post-partum depression. Front Neurosci 13:833. https://doi.org/10.3389/fnins.2019.00833

Picard M, Scott-Boyer M-P, Bodein A et al (2021) Integration strategies of multi-omics data for machine learning analysis. Comput Struct Biotechnol J 19:3735–3746. https://doi.org/10.1016/j.csbj.2021.06.030

Ritchie MD, Holzinger ER, Li R et al (2015) Methods of integrating data to uncover genotype–phenotype interactions. Nat Rev Genet 16:85–97. https://doi.org/10.1038/nrg3868

Rolland AD, Evrard B, Darde TA et al (2019) RNA profiling of human testicular cells identifies syntenic lncRNAs associated with spermatogenesis. Hum Reprod 34:1278–1290. https://doi.org/10.1093/humrep/dez063

Romero R, Yeo L, Miranda J et al (2013) A blueprint for the prevention of preterm birth: vaginal progesterone in women with a short cervix. J Perinat Med 41:27–44. https://doi.org/10.1515/jpm-2012-0272

Sriboonvorakul N, Hu J, Boriboonhirunsarn D et al (2022) Proteomics studies in gestational diabetes mellitus: a systematic review and meta-analysis. JCM 11:2737. https://doi.org/10.3390/jcm11102737

Sung H, Ferlay J, Siegel RL et al (2021) Global cancer statistics 2020: GLOBOCAN estimates of incidence and mortality worldwide for 36 cancers in 185 countries. CA A Cancer J Clin 71:209–249. https://doi.org/10.3322/caac.21660

Tarazona S, Arzalluz-Luque A, Conesa A (2021) Undisclosed, unmet and neglected challenges in multi-omics studies. Nat Comput Sci 1:395–402. https://doi.org/10.1038/s43588-021-00086-z

Tarca AL, Pataki BÁ, Romero R et al (2021) Crowdsourcing assessment of maternal blood multi-omics for predicting gestational age and preterm birth. Cell Rep Med 2:100323. https://doi.org/10.1016/j.xcrm.2021.100323

Tebani A, Afonso C, Marret S, Bekri S (2016) Omics-based strategies in precision medicine: toward a paradigm shift in inborn errors of metabolism investigations. IJMS 17:1555. https://doi.org/10.3390/ijms17091555

Vellido A (2019) Societal issues concerning the application of artificial intelligence in medicine. Kidney Dis 5:11–17. https://doi.org/10.1159/000492428

Wang S-W, Ma L-L, Huang S et al (2016) Role of cervical cerclage and vaginal progesterone in the treatment of cervical incompetence with/without preterm birth history. Chin Med J 129:2670–2675. https://doi.org/10.4103/0366-6999.193451

Xiao Y, Bi M, Guo H, Li M (2022) Multi-omics approaches for biomarker discovery in early ovarian cancer diagnosis. EBioMedicine 79:104001. https://doi.org/10.1016/j.ebiom.2022.104001

Yu Y, Liang H-F, Chen J et al (2021) Postpartum depression: current status and possible identification using biomarkers. Front Psych 12:620371. https://doi.org/10.3389/fpsyt.2021.620371

Zeng H, Chen L, Zhang M et al (2021) Integration of histopathological images and multi-dimensional omics analyses predicts molecular features and prognosis in high-grade serous ovarian cancer. Gynecol Oncol 163:171–180. https://doi.org/10.1016/j.ygyno.2021.07.015

Zhang P-Y, Yu Y (2020) Precise personalized medicine in gynecology cancer and infertility. Front Cell Dev Biol 7:382. https://doi.org/10.3389/fcell.2019.00382

Zhang L, Zou W, Huang Y et al (2019a) A preliminary study of uric metabolomic alteration for postpartum depression based on liquid chromatography coupled to quadrupole time-of-flight mass spectrometry. Dis Markers 2019:1–9. https://doi.org/10.1155/2019/4264803

Zhang X, Zhang P, Song D et al (2019b) Expression profiles and characteristics of human lncRNA in normal and asthenozoospermia sperm†. Biol Reprod 100:982–993. https://doi.org/10.1093/biolre/ioy253

Zhang L, Zheng Q, Xie H et al (2020) Quantitative cervical elastography: a new approach of cervical insufficiency prediction. Arch Gynecol Obstet 301:207–215. https://doi.org/10.1007/s00404-019-05377-5

Zhou X, Chai H, Zhao H et al (2020) Imputing missing RNA-sequencing data from DNA methylation by using a transfer learning–based neural network. GigaScience 9:giaa076. https://doi.org/10.1093/gigascience/giaa076

Association Rule Mining in Reproductive Health Data

5

Srishti Verma, Vishal, Keshav Mittal, Muskan Syed,
Payal Gupta, Gaurav Majumdar, and Priyanka Narad

Abstract

The goal of the chapter is to understand the concept of association rule mining (ARM) which a fundamental data mining technique is crucial for uncovering patterns and dependencies in large datasets, particularly in the context of reproductive health. This chapter focuses on identifying the order explaining co-occurrences or dependencies among significant data points, creating "if-then" association statements. Further, the chapter uses the concept of transactions representing sets of items observed together such as ARM factors like clinical conditions, treatment modalities, lifestyle choices, and demographic attributes. The chapter outlines the techniques that aid in extracting actionable insights from complex datasets encompassing electronic medical records, gene expression data, medical imaging records, and clinical data sources. The chapter explains the process which begins with data identification, collection, and preprocessing to ensure quality and privacy. The chapter further hypothesizes that ARM algorithms will unveil actionable patterns for healthcare practitioners and researchers, such as the impact of treatments on reproductive outcomes or associations between lifestyle factors and fertility.

S. Verma · Vishal · K. Mittal · M. Syed · P. Gupta
Systems Biology and Data Analytics Research Lab, Amity Institute of Biotechnology, Amity University, Uttar Pradesh, Noida, India

G. Majumdar
Centre of IVF and Human Reproduction, Sir Ganga Ram Hospital, New Delhi, India

P. Narad (✉)
Division of Biomedical Informatics (BMI), Indian Council of Medical Research, New Delhi, India

A. Sengupta et al. (eds.), *Data-Driven Reproductive Health*,
https://doi.org/10.1007/978-981-97-7451-7_5

Keywords

Association rule mining · Reproductive health · Apriori algorithm · Family planning · Prenatal care

5.1 Introduction

Association rule mining is a fundamental data mining technique aimed at uncovering interesting patterns, dependencies, and relationships inherent in large datasets. At its center, this methodology aims to identify the order that explains the co-occurrence or dependencies between different significant data points in a dataset, forming an "if-then" association statement. Transactions, representing sets of items bought or observed together, form the basis of analysis. In the context of reproductive health, this resonates with the exploration of the association between numerous factors such as clinical conditions, treatment modalities, lifestyle choices, and demographic attributes. In this method, two key metrics, support, and confidence, quantify the frequency of item set occurrence and reliability of association rules, respectively. ARM technique has found substantial implementation in the context of reproductive health, reproductive health encompasses a broad spectrum of medical and healthcare considerations, ranging from fertility, and family planning to prenatal care, childbirth, and post-natal healthcare (Yazgana and Kusakci 2016). Within this complex domain, the utilization of ARM becomes pivotal for gleaning actionable insights from intricate datasets, consisting of electronic medical records, gene expression data, medical imaging records, medical histories, and other clinical data sources.

The mining process typically begins with the identification and collection of relevant data, which can include clinical data, medical histories, omics data, diagnostic codes, treatment plans, and demographic details. Ensuring the quality, integrity, and privacy of this data is paramount. Subsequently, preprocessing steps are undertaken to clean and transform the raw data into a suitable format for analysis. This involves handling missing values, standardizing data formats, and encoding categorical variables. The prepared dataset is then subjected to the ARM algorithms, with the Apriori algorithm being one of the most employed techniques, this algorithm identifies frequent item set, which are sets of items that often appear together in the dataset, and generates association rules based on user-defined metrics such as support and confidence. Support, the context of ARM, refers to the proportion of records in the dataset that contain a specific data point. High support indicates that the data point is prevalent in the data. Confidence, on the other hand, measures the likelihood that the associated item in a rule will occur given the antecedent item set. In the end, a high-confidence rule suggests a strong association between the antecedent and the consequent. ARM is applied to address various research questions

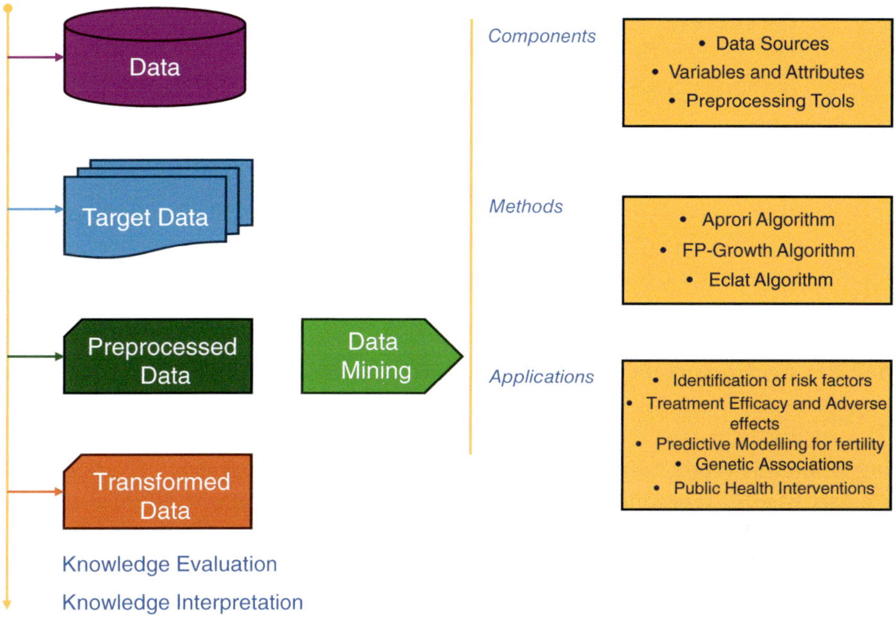

Fig. 5.1 Knowledge discovery/interpretation in association rule mining. The workflow further illustrates the process of association rule mining, encompassing data collection, preprocessing, transformation, and analysis. It features components like data sources and variables, preprocessing tools, and methods such as the Apriori, FP-growth, and Eclat algorithms, culminating in diverse applications across domains

and solve healthcare challenges, the most common of which exploring comorbidity among reproductive health conditions, helping researchers and clinicians anticipate potential complications and condition overlapping. Figure 5.1 demonstrates the knowledge discovery/interpretation in association rule mining and its associated workflow.

The integration of ARM findings with reproductive healthcare practices holds immense promise. Researchers and healthcare practitioners can leverage discovered associations to tailor interventions, enhance diagnostic accuracy, and optimize treatment plans. The synthesis of findings from this process in reproductive health is dynamic, involving the identification of associations and the interpretation of their clinical significance. The study hypothesizes that the utilization of ARM algorithms will uncover patterns that can be translated into actionable knowledge for healthcare practitioners and researchers. These patterns include the co-occurrence of specific medical conditions, the impact of certain treatments on reproductive outcomes, or the association between lifestyle factors and fertility.

5.2 Overview

5.2.1 Introduction

The chapter starts by introducing the field of association rule mining about reproductive health. It shows the importance of studying concealed patterns and links among various datasets on reproductive health. This introduction is about complicated data concerning reproduction that includes genetic, clinical, and lifestyle factors that necessitate sophisticated analytic techniques.

5.2.2 Components of Association Rule Mining

This section explains the main parts of the process involved in association rule mining within the reproductive health context. It provides an overview of various data sources used in reproductive health datasets, with emphasis on variables such as patient demographics, genetic markers, and medical history. The discussion also covers preprocessing tools important for cleaning and converting data into a format suitable for analysis.

5.2.3 Methods of Association Rule Mining

Reproductive health databases have many complex relationships which are usually decoded by association rule mining. This method comprises Apriori, FP-Growth, and Eclat algorithms that bring out patterns between genetic markers, lifestyle factors, and reproductive outcomes. Genetic algorithm-based approaches optimize the search for intricate relationships while temporal mining captures evolving variables from preconception to postpartum (Kaushik et al. 2021). Geographical influences are considered in spatial mining that further reveal region-specific patterns and environmental factors affecting fertility outcomes. Hybridizing association rule mining with predictive modeling provides a comprehensive view of reproductive health data. Consequently, healthcare professionals get empowered and can make decisions based on informed choices, create better interventions, and improve overall reproductive health outcomes. Association rule mining offers a nuanced perspective on reproductive health data, contributing to an enhanced understanding of factors affecting fertility, genetic predisposition, and maternal health.

5.2.4 Applications in Reproductive Health

Association rule mining is applicable in many reproductive health issues; thus, the approach was changed by how medical practitioners deal with fertility, maternal well-being, and genetic aspects. Providing preconception care identifies patterns of lifestyle that affect fertility and allows for personalized interventions for parents before they conceive. In pregnancy, it discovers connections between expectant mothers' activities, environmental factors, and birth outcomes hence helping to target precise prenatal care tactics. It is used to gain insights into postnatal complications and optimize post-delivery care plans. This method helps find complicated relationships between genetic markers and reproductive disorders, thus understanding possible hereditary dispositions. It improves the decision-making processes involving ART by unraveling factors influencing its success rates. Geographical applications enable the identification of regional disparities in reproductive health necessitating policymakers' design of place-specific interventions.

5.2.5 Objective of This Study

The chapter then explicitly outlines the overarching objective of conducting an association rule mining study in reproductive health. It emphasizes the aim to unveil hidden associations, discover novel risk factors, and optimize treatment strategies. The hypothesis is hinted at, indicating a focus on improving predictive models for fertility outcomes based on the extracted associations. This section clarifies the research goals and provides a roadmap for the ensuing sections.

5.2.6 Detailed Explanation of Association Rules

This chapter provides a detailed explanation of association rules concerning reproductive health data. It dissects the concept, elucidates the parameters involved, and provides a nuanced understanding of how these rules manifest in the intricate landscape of reproductive health datasets. Real-world scenarios and examples may be incorporated for enhanced clarity.

5.2.7 Conclusion

The chapter concludes with a summary that recalls the major ideas and preparations for the next section. It underscores the relevance of association rule mining to improving our understanding of issues of reproduction health and intimate's wider clinical implications for medical practitioners, researchers, and policymakers.

5.2.8 Applications in Reproductive Medicine: Transforming Lives and Families

Reproductive medicine has embarked on a transformative journey, offering hope and solutions to individuals and couples navigating fertility challenges. This dynamic field encompasses a range of therapies that enhance reproductive function, promote safe pregnancies, and enable individuals to make educated decisions regarding their reproductive health. It goes beyond simple conception facilitation (Smith et al. 2016). This paper delves into some transformative applications within this field and highlights their impact through vivid examples.

5.3 Assisted Reproductive Technologies (ART)

The advent of ART has unlocked new avenues for family building. In vitro fertilization (IVF) stands as the cornerstone, bypassing natural obstacles by fertilizing eggs and sperm outside the body. The resultant embryos are then carefully cultivated and inserted into the uterus, providing a lifeline to couples experiencing severe male factor infertility, endometriosis, or obstructed fallopian tubes. This technology has empowered countless individuals to experience parenthood, diagnosed with female and male factor infertility (Kushnir et al. 2022).

Beyond IVF, advancements extend to intracytoplasmic sperm injection (ICSI) and gamete cryopreservation. ICSI offers a beacon of hope for couples burdened with severe male infertility by directly injecting a single sperm into an egg, bypassing issues like low sperm count or motility (Neri et al. 2014). This technique allows both the carriers of a genetic condition, to have a healthy child free of the disease through IVF with preimplantation genetic diagnosis (PGD). Meanwhile, cryopreservation empowers individuals facing medical treatments like chemotherapy or those choosing delayed childbearing to preserve their eggs, sperm, or embryos for future use. Imagine a female young cancer patient, undergoing egg freezing before treatment; this technology protects her future ability to experience motherhood on her terms.

5.3.1 Preimplantation Genetic Testing (PGT)

PGT has emerged as a meaningful change in fertility care, providing an invaluable tool for couples facing specific genetic risks or a history of recurrent pregnancy loss. By analyzing the genetic makeup of embryos before implantation, PGT offers invaluable information about their viability and potential for healthy development (Fesahat et al. 2020). For example, PGT-A pinpoints chromosomal abnormalities like aneuploidy, a primary cause of miscarriage and birth defects. This technology allows both male and female carriers of cystic fibrosis, to select genetically healthy embryos for transfer, significantly reducing the risk of passing the condition on to their children.

Furthermore, PGT-M/N diagnoses specific monogenic disorders, carriers of Tay-Sachs disease, to make informed decisions about embryo selection and prevent the transmission of this devastating condition. The impact of PGT extends beyond genetic disorders; it can also identify embryos with the most potential for successful implantation, optimizing pregnancy outcomes and minimizing the emotional and financial burden of multiple IVF cycles (Wang et al. 2019). This personalized approach revolutionizes fertility care, empowering couples with valuable information to make informed choices about their family-building journey.

5.3.2 Minimally Invasive Surgery (MIS)

The era of extensive surgical procedures in reproductive medicine is giving way to the burgeoning field of minimally invasive surgery (MIS) (Hamad and Curet 2010). Laparoscopic and robotic surgeries offer a change in basic assumptions in treating conditions like endometriosis, fibroids, and pelvic adhesions, previously managed through larger incisions. These techniques utilize delicate instruments inserted through tiny keyhole incisions, minimizing tissue damage, reducing pain, and shortening recovery times.

Take the case of a female patient, diagnosed with severe endometriosis causing debilitating pain and infertility. Traditional surgery would have left her with large scars and a lengthy recovery period. However, thanks to MIS, she can undergo a successful laparoscopic endometriosis ablation, experiencing minimal pain. This transformative approach not only minimizes physical discomfort but also reduces emotional stress and allows patients to resume their lives quickly.

Robotic surgery further elevates the MIS experience by offering enhanced precision and dexterity. A patient diagnosed with large uterine fibroids that were previously deemed inoperable due to their complex location. Through robotic myomectomy, the surgeon could navigate the intricate anatomy with unparalleled precision, removing the fibroids successfully with minimal blood loss and tissue damage. This technology expands the surgical options for complex cases, offering hope to patients who were previously considered inoperable.

5.4 Preparation and Preprocessing

5.4.1 Introduction to Preprocessing

The introduction to preprocessing in the domain of reproductive health data is a crucial step when preparing datasets for association rule mining. In the complex landscape of reproductive health, preprocessing plays a crucial role in refining raw data. Noise elimination, anomaly rectification, and maintaining data homogeneity are among the functions of it that set the stage for extracting meaningful patterns. Reproductive health datasets entail demographic details and medical histories among other information sources presenting challenges such as missing values and outliers. Consequently, neglecting these issues may compromise subsequent analysis. For this reason, researchers employ advanced data-cleaning methods that consider the effects of each decision on the integrity of the analysis itself.

Temporality is a critical consideration when dealing with reproductive health data due to its dynamic nature over time. The introduction chapter on preprocessing discusses techniques designed for handling these temporal dimensions by emphasizing capturing dynamic patterns within an analytical framework. In reproductive health data privacy aspect is very delicate and therefore researchers must be careful in securing patients' sensitive information. Preprocessing emphasizes the need to prepare raw data for association rule mining algorithms, where the success of subsequent analysis depends on the accuracy applied during this preparation phase. As researchers navigate this maze, they assume the role of the alchemist, transforming raw data into knowledge through a crucible of preprocessing.

5.4.2 Data Cleaning and Filtering

In the context of reproductive health, the process of data cleansing and filtering is the foundation for preparing datasets for association code mining. The importance of clean datasets in the complex field of reproductive health research cannot be overstated. This phase involves identifying and correcting common issues such as missing values, outliers, and errors, which can significantly affect the reliability of subsequent analyses. Purifying data is like purifying raw materials before gaining valuable insights (Prasad et al. 2011). Researchers should handle missing values with caution and ensure that data gaps are filled appropriately to avoid biased interpretations. Outstanding indicators of gaps or errors must be judiciously identified and corrected to prevent distortions in the dataset that could compromise the integrity of findings This nuanced process requires clarity love in context and domain-specific knowledge of reproductive health issues.

Filtering is a parallel but separate element of this preparatory stage. Involving selective retention or exclusion of data according to some criteria that would ensure the dataset is tailored to the specific requirements of reproductive health analysis. Filtering can mean selecting only relevant variables, periods, or subsets of data that fit into the research focus. This strategic curation enhances dataset relevance and reduces noise, facilitating more focused and meaningful investigation for associations.

The interplay between data cleaning and filtering is crucial for a refined dataset. Cleaning involves addressing missing values and anomalies while filtering assists a researcher to choose which parts of the data may add most value to association rule mining process. This tandem approach resembles making an artist's masterpiece where every stroke helps refine raw material to arrive at a shape that will encourage the discovery of meaningful patterns within reproductive health data. In conclusion, data cleaning and filtering are the foundation of preparing datasets for association like mining in reproductive health.

5.4.3 Discretization of Continuous Variables

Discretization is a key stage in preparing datasets for association rule mining and is applied to continuous variables in reproductive health data. Mining algorithms are faced with a significant problem when it comes to working with continuous variables, which usually have a range of values (Muhlenbach and Rakotomalala 2005). The process involves transforming these variables from continuous to discrete groups or bins that enable the identification of patterns.

In reproductive health, most variables such as age, hormone levels, and cycle durations are often continuous hence discretization should be done. Some common methods include clustering and binning splitting up the continuous ranges into separate categories. This not only suits algorithmic tastes but also makes interpretation easier thereby helping to identify meaningful associations within the data. Choosing the discretization method is critical. The nature of the data should be well thought-out before choosing an approach as well as being aware of association rule mining's requirement for carrying out analysis. Optimal discretization helps in capturing reproductive health-related patterns thus providing deeper insights during future analysis.

In other words, it can be said that discretization constitutes a way of aligning association rule mining towards reproductive health data. By converting continuous variables into discrete categories, researchers pave the way for more effective pattern recognition and interpretation, contributing to a nuanced understanding of reproductive health dynamics.

5.4.4 Categorical Variable Encoding

When it comes to association rule mining, categorical variable encoding is key in preparing the reproductive health data for meticulousness, serving as a link between the categorical nature of information and the numerical requirements of mining algorithms (Uyar et al. 2009). Reproductive health research is a vast field that relies heavily on categorical variables such as patient condition, medical treatment, or diagnostic categories; hence, encoding becomes important for efficient pattern extraction and association discovery.

5.4.4.1 Significance of Categorical Variable Encoding

Categorical variables play a crucial role in reproductive health datasets, as they represent discrete states or classes. Nevertheless, most association rule mining algorithms are designed to work with numerical data. The seamless integration of categorical variable encoding is therefore imperative to enable the algorithms to identify patterns within the data.

5.4.4.2 Encoding Techniques

Categorical variable encoding employs two main techniques: hot encoding and label encoding. With one-hot encoding, each category is transformed into a binary feature resulting in a binary matrix representation. Label encoding assigns numeric labels to categories thus creating a numerical mapping for algorithmic processing. The choice between these techniques depends on such factors as the nature of the data and the particular requirements of association rule mining algorithms.

5.4.4.3 Algorithmic Suitability

The appropriateness of encoding techniques is closely associated with the concepts applied in association rule mining. One-hot encoding usually retains independence among classes by disregarding any order among categories. In contrast, label encoding may be helpful if there is an order between categories. Thus, reproductive health data should be encoded using specific techniques that will make it compatible with mining algorithms for accurate and relevant associations.

5.4.4.4 Enhanced Interpretation

Categorical variable encoding is crucial in maintaining the interpretability of reproductive health data besides algorithmic compatibility. Encoded variables retain their categorical meaning even when algorithms process numerical representations to ensure that insights from association rule mining are algorithmically sound and clinically meaningful.

Indeed, categorical variable encoding proves to be a transformational strategy towards gaining valuable insights from reproductive health data. It allows numerical representation of categorical variables, which not only adhere to operational requirements of association rule mining algorithms but also enhance the interpretability of discovered patterns enabling a more comprehensive understanding of reproductive health dynamics.

5.5 Feature Scaling

Feature scaling is a crucial step in preparing reproductive health data for association rule mining. It entails converting numerical features to a common scale, ensuring that variables of varying magnitudes contribute equally to the mining process (Wan 2019). In reproductive health, where variables such as hormone levels or patient ages might vary, feature scaling improves the performance of mining algorithms by avoiding biases generated by disparate scales and facilitating more accurate pattern recognition and connection finding.

5.6 Documentation of Preprocessing Steps: Ensuring Methodological Transparency and Analytical Reproducibility

In the intricate tapestry of association rule mining applied to reproductive health data, meticulous documentation of preprocessing steps stands as a beacon of methodological rigor and analytical trustworthiness. The journey of documentation unfolds through several imperative steps, each contributing to the clarity and precision of the research process.

5.6.1 Record of Initial Dataset Dynamics

The first thing to do in the process of documentation is to capture some essential information about the origin of the raw dataset, dimension and how variables relate. It is called foundational step because this helps provide a framework that will be used in subsequent data preprocessing moves.

5.6.2 Transparent Account of Data Cleaning Procedures

It should deal with the technicalities involved in ensuring that data is cleaned by explaining how missing values were filled, outliers detected, and errors rectified. This step acts as the sentinel for data integrity as it strengthens it against probable biases and distortions.

5.6.3 Criteria-Driven Data Filtering Chronicles

It should unveil specific temporal segments or variables determining whether they are included or excluded from any given datasets. In this way, one can get an insight into how the researcher curated the dataset strategically, thereby distilling it to its essence.

5.6.4 In-Depth Exploration of Discretization and Encoding Strategies

This layer of documentation will reveal all aspects involving categorizing continuous variables and encoding categorical counterpart elements. The raw heterogeneous forms of such datasets make up the methodological alchemy employed to transform them into digestible forms upon which mining algorithms are applicable with care.

5.6.5 Temporal Nuances and Privacy Safeguards in Focus

The documentation should show us how time was cleverly weaved into preprocessing actions; while at the same time protecting confidential information and outlining measures taken to anonymize and aggregate data, a testament to the commitment to ethical data handling.

5.6.6 Numerical Harmony Through Feature Scaling Description

Prepare to penetrate the realm of numbers as feature scaling reconciles different magnitudes. Highlight the chosen scaling approach and its effect on algorithmic efficiency and quality of the analytical lens.

5.6.7 Summation in a Final Dataset Manifesto

Complete the documentation journey by summarizing the final dataset which is an overview of what has been done in preprocessing. This report is a foundational pillar for data transparency that provides insight into critical attributes of transformed data so that other researchers can apply this information in their work.

The documentation of preprocessing steps, moving beyond a mere procedural account, transcends into a statement about the researcher's commitment to analytical excellence. It tells a story that not only strengthens the integrity within but also opens it up externally making it more prone to criticism, thus reinforcing the basic principles of scholarly debate and bolstering the overall fabric of knowledge about reproductive health.

5.7 Future Directions and Challenges in Preprocessing for Association Rule Mining in Reproductive Health Data: Paving the Way Forward

As we navigate the evolving landscape of preprocessing in association rule mining for reproductive health data, several promising avenues beckon, accompanied by nuanced challenges that demand attention. This brief exploration lays the foundation for future endeavors.

5.7.1 Future Directions

5.7.1.1 Integration of Advanced Machine Learning Techniques

To explore synergies between preprocessing and advanced machine learning techniques, increasing the adaptability of algorithms to unique intricacies of reproductive health data.

5.7.1.2 Dynamic Preprocessing Frameworks

Develop frameworks that can dynamically adjust their preprocessing steps based on changing data patterns such that they are stable in case there is any temporal fluctuation.

5.7.1.3 Enhanced Privacy-Preserving Measures

Innovate privacy-preserving methods that balance data utility with patient confidentiality, thus increasing trust and compliance in a time when data privacy is a major concern.

5.8 Challenges

5.8.1 Handling Increasing Data Volume and Complexity

Deal with rising volumes and increasingly complicated reproductive health data through new preprocessing methods capable of dealing with the increased dimensions of datasets.

5.8.2 Ethical Dilemmas in Data Utilization

Tackle ethical complexities of data manipulation by finding ways to draw insights from data while at the same time ensuring that the rights and private lives of those contributing to research on reproductive health are preserved.

5.8.3 Interdisciplinary Collaboration Gaps

Overcome interdisciplinary barriers through partnerships between data scientists, healthcare professionals, and ethicists as a way of aligning preprocessing in reproductive healthcare processes.

Finally, the future of preprocessing toward association rule mining reproductive health data still holds hope for transformative advancements. Simultaneously, the challenges underscore the imperative for a meticulous, ethical, and collaborative approach, setting the stage for a dynamic and impactful trajectory in this vital domain.

5.9 Mining Association Rules in Reproductive Dataset

5.9.1 Association Rules

Association rules represent conditional statements that uncover relationships within diverse datasets, such as those found in a reproductive health dataset. In the context of reproductive health, these rules serve as invaluable tools to discern intricate patterns and connections within patient data. Leveraging if/then statements, association rules unveil dependencies between unrelated variables, contributing to a nuanced understanding of factors influencing reproductive health outcomes. The application of association rules in reproductive health data is multifaceted. It extends beyond traditional uses, encompassing basket data analysis, classification, cross-marketing, clustering, catalog design, and loss-leader analysis. For instance, if a patient has been diagnosed with a specific reproductive health condition, association rules might reveal a higher likelihood of co-occurring conditions or suggest correlated factors influencing health outcomes.

Consider an example: if a patient has a history of polycystic ovary syndrome (PCOS), association rules may unveil a significant association with insulin resistance or hormonal imbalances. This information can guide healthcare professionals in devising more targeted and personalized treatment plans.

Two pivotal criteria, support, and confidence, form the backbone of association rules in reproductive health datasets. Support quantifies the frequency of a particular association, measuring how often a given pattern occurs. On the other hand, confidence gauges the association's reliability, indicating the probability that the consequent variable will occur given the antecedent variable.

$$\text{Support}\left(A \Rightarrow B\right) = \frac{\text{Freq}\left(A,B\right)}{N}$$

$$\text{Confidence}\left(A \Rightarrow B\right) = \frac{\text{Freq}\left(A,B\right)}{\text{Freq}\left(A\right)}$$

5.9.2 AIS Algorithm

When it comes to association rule mining, the AIS (Agrawal, Imielinski, and Swami) method is considered a foundational addition to the area, especially when used with reproductive health datasets. Agrawal, Imielinski, and Swami sought to use the essential features of this algorithm to improve database quality and aid in decision-making. AIS is unique in that it generates association rules with just one-item consequents, such as $X \cap Y \Rightarrow Z$ rather than $X \Rightarrow Y \cap Z$.

Within the algorithm, the process of extracting meaningful insights from the reproductive health dataset involves multiple scans to derive frequent data point sets (Zhao and Bhowmick 2003). The initial pass across the dataset focuses on aggregating the support count for each data point. This count is crucial, as it forms the basis for subsequent decisions. Data points failing to meet the specified minimal support count are strategically excluded from the list, streamlining the dataset for meaningful analysis (Khurana 2013).

In the algorithm, data points with high frequency were generated by iterating over the database several times, during the earlier iterations the support count for the data points was accumulated. Data points with a support count below the threshold are removed from the data window, subsequently, a new data window is formed by extending frequent data points with other transaction items. In the second pass, the support count of these candidate data points is accumulated and compared to the support threshold. This process continues, generating candidate (k + 1)-data points by extending a frequent k-item set with transaction items. The iteration persists until either the candidate item sets or the frequent item sets become empty.

The AIS algorithm's limitation becomes more pronounced (Ish Nath Jha 2013). The algorithm's drawback lies in the generation of an excessive number of candidate data points, which prove to be small when applied to reproductive data. This overgeneration results in increased space requirements and wasted computational effort. In the specific domain of reproductive datasets, where the data may already be voluminous and complex, the algorithm's propensity to create numerous candidate data points can lead to inefficient use of resources. Furthermore, the algorithm demands multiple passes over the entire reproductive database, intensifying the computational burden. Given the sensitive nature of reproductive data and the potential intricacies involved, the requirement for repeated scans exacerbates concerns related to both time and resource utilization. This increased demand for computational resources may pose challenges, especially in scenarios where efficiency and expediency are crucial considerations.

5.9.3 SETM Algorithm

In the SETM algorithm, prospective data points are dynamically generated while scanning the reproductive dataset, with actual counting deferred until the conclusion of the pass. The subsequent creation of new candidate data points mirrors the process in the AIS algorithm, with an additional step (Kerana Hanirex and Kaliyamurthie 2016). In this method, the patient identifier of the generating transaction is preserved alongside the candidate data point within a sequential structure. This strategic separation of the candidate generation from the counting process is a distinctive feature. Upon completing the pass, the support count of candidate data points is determined by consolidating the information stored in the sequential structure.

Despite its efficacy, the SETM algorithm shares a drawback with the AIS algorithm. An additional limitation is evident in the extensive entries associated with each candidate data point, equating to its support value. This redundancy poses a challenge in terms of computational efficiency and storage requirements, highlighting a notable disadvantage of the SETM algorithm within the context of reproductive health datasets.

5.10 Apriori Algorithm

The Apriori algorithm is a widely employed technique in the realm of reproductive health data analysis (Yuan 2017). The algorithm plays a crucial role in identifying recurring patterns and associations within datasets related to reproductive health. Like its application in frequent pattern mining (FPM) for general datasets, the Apriori algorithm is instrumental in discovering regularities and relationships between various aspects of reproductive health data. Reproductive health data often involves the identification of recurring patterns or relationships between different health indicators. Frequent pattern mining in this context entails the exploration of sets of health indicators or item set that frequently co-occur in each dataset. These recurring sets termed frequent patterns, are gauged by the frequency of their occurrence across multiple instances, such as patient records or specific periods.

5.10.1 Components of Apriori Algorithm

$$\text{Support}(A) = \frac{\text{Number of Transactions in which } A \text{ occurs}}{\text{Numbers of all Transactions}}$$

$$\text{Lift}(A \to B) = \frac{\text{Support}(A \text{ and } B)}{\text{Support}(A).\text{Support}(B)}$$

$$\text{Confidence}(A \Rightarrow B) = P\left(\frac{B}{A}\right) = \frac{(A \cup B)}{(A)}$$

5.10.2 Steps in Apriori Algorithm

The steps of association rule mining using the Apriori algorithm involve several essential steps (Fig. 5.2). Starting with, defining the minimum support threshold, representing the minimum frequency of an item set must have in the dataset to be considered frequent (Hegland 2007). This threshold is based on the dataset's size and domain knowledge. Following this, a list of one-item set is generated by iterating over the entire dataset and identifying the items that meet the minimum support criteria. In the next step, the algorithm progresses to generate C_k set by creating a list of sets with a length of K + 1 from the frequent K-item sets used in the previous set. Again, the support of each candidate item set is counted by iterating over the dataset once again. After each iteration, the candidate item set that does not meet the minimum support threshold is pruned from the consideration of the algorithm. This process of generating candidate item sets, calculating threshold, and pruning continues until no more frequent item sets can be generated.

5.10.3 Limitations

The computational complexity of the Apriori algorithm leads to challenges especially when applied to large reproductive health datasets characterized by substantial sample size. For example, a dataset featuring a count of frequent one-item sets, such as 10^4 will generate more than 10^7 two-item set candidates making the algorithm computationally burdensome. Also, the algorithm's tendency to produce many rules can impede the efficient identification of crucial patterns within reproductive health data. Moreover, the algorithm's reliance on multiple dataset iterations may act as a limiting factor where access to data is slow and expensive, hindering the practicality of reproductive health information systems.

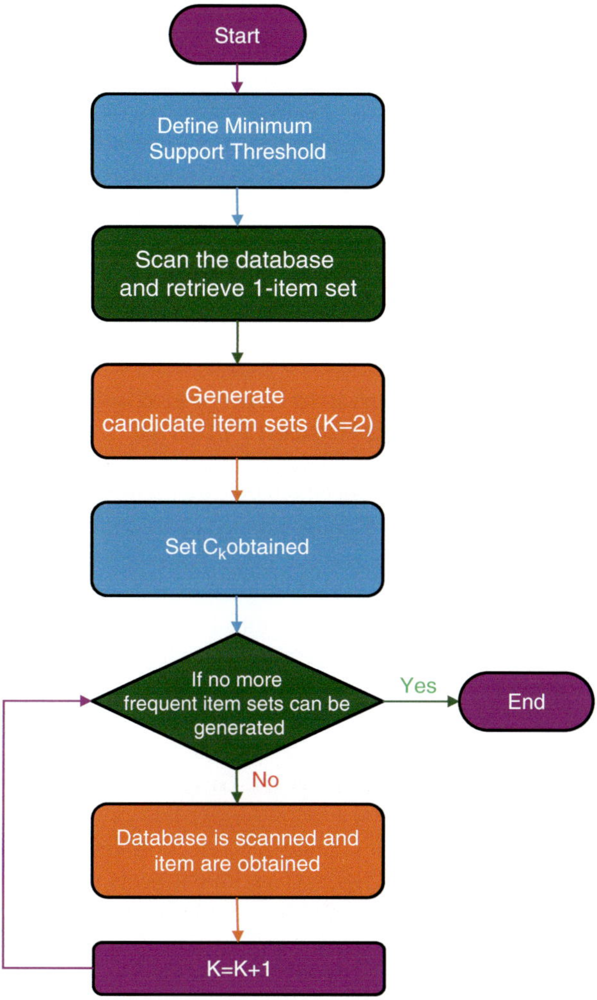

Fig. 5.2 Detailed workflow for the Apriori algorithm, a pivotal method in association rule mining. It delineates key steps, including setting the minimum support threshold, scanning the database to retrieve item sets, generating candidate item sets, and iteratively pruning infrequent item sets. This systematic approach ensures efficient discovery of meaningful associations within the dataset, contributing to insightful knowledge extraction and analysis

5.11 FP-Growth Algorithm

To address the drawbacks of the Apriori algorithm, the FP-growth algorithm proves to be a valuable alternative. Overcoming the challenges of multiple database iterations and candidate generation. The FP-growth algorithm employs a divide-and-conquer strategy, requiring only two passes over the dataset (Zhang et al. 2008).

In the first pass, the algorithm conducts a comprehensive analysis, computing a list of frequent data points sorted by their frequencies in descending order, known as the F-list. Simultaneously, the algorithm scans the dataset to discover and discard the infrequent data points, optimizing the process. The frequent items are then sorted based on their support, constructing the foundation for the generation of the

FP-tree. The order established during this sorting step allows the creation of the FP-tree, facilitating the sharing of common prefixes and enhancing efficiency.

In the second pass, the FP-tree is utilized to perform the mining recursively. Modes within the tree represent data points, each equipped with a counter. As FP-growth reads one transaction at a time, it maps the transaction to a path within the tree. A fixed order is established, ensuring that paths can overlap when transactions share common data points. The data point counters are incremented accordingly, and pointers are established between the nodes containing the same data point, creating a singly linked list. The more paths that overlap, the higher the compression achieved by the FP-tree, making it memory efficient.

5.12 Evaluation and Interpretation of Association Rules: Unveiling Hidden Patterns

Unearthing valuable insights from vast datasets is the cornerstone of data mining, and association rule mining (ARM) plays a crucial role in this endeavor. However, simply generating numerous rules from data is insufficient; robust evaluation and insightful interpretation are key to extracting genuine knowledge and actionable insights. This section delves into the essential metrics for evaluating association rules and explores effective techniques for gleaning their true meaning, empowering researchers and data analysts to navigate the world of ARM with confidence.

5.12.1 Evaluation Metrics: Guiding the Light

A plethora of metrics guide the selection and interpretation of association rules. These metrics shed light on various aspects of a rule's relevance and usefulness, ensuring that researchers focus on rules with genuine implications (Bao et al. 2021). Here are some of the most crucial evaluation metrics.

5.12.2 Support

Measuring the prevalence of an item set, support reflects how frequently a rule's antecedent and consequent occur together within the data. A rule with high support indicates a common pattern, while a low support rule may represent a niche phenomenon.

5.12.3 Confidence

Quantifying the reliability of a rule, confidence expresses how often the consequence occurs given the presence of the antecedent. A high-confidence rule suggests a strong association between the item sets, whereas a low-confidence rule warns against drawing firm conclusions.

5.12.4 Lift

Assessing the unexpectedness of a rule, lift compares the observed association with the probability of occurrence by chance. A lift value greater than 1 indicates a pattern deviating from random chance, signifying a potentially valuable rule.

5.12.5 Conviction

Evaluating the direction of the association, conviction measures the ratio of the confidence for the original rule to the confidence for its inverse. A conviction value greater than 1 strengthens the directionality of the rule, while a value less than 1 suggests caution in interpreting the causal link.

5.12.6 Interestingness Measures

Beyond quantitative metrics, subjective measures like novelty, unexpectedness, and actionability contribute to rule selection. These measures capture the human element of rule evaluation, ensuring that chosen rules spark deeper investigation and lead to actionable insights.

5.13 Interpretation Techniques: Demystifying the Code

Evaluating a rule is just the first step; extracting its true meaning is crucial for knowledge-building and practical applications. Various interpretation techniques delve into the complexities of an association rule, revealing its context and potential implications (Yedjour and Benyettou 2018). Here are some prominent techniques.

5.13.1 Domain Knowledge Integration

Grounding the interpretation in domain expertise adds context and meaning to the identified patterns. Researchers should leverage their understanding of the specific domain to explain the relationships between item sets and draw relevant conclusions.

5.13.2 Visualizations

Employing visual representations like bar charts, heat maps, and network diagrams can enhance the comprehension of associations. Visualizing the data can reveal hidden patterns, outliers, and clusters, providing deeper insights into the relationships between variables.

5.13.3 Rule Clustering

Grouping similar rules based on shared characteristics allows for efficient analysis and interpretation. Clustering helps identify broader trends and patterns in the data, reducing the complexity of interpreting numerous individual rules.

5.13.4 Rule Reframing

Rephrasing rules in natural language or using case studies can improve their accessibility and interpretability for non-technical audiences. This facilitates communication and collaboration, ensuring that valuable insights reach stakeholders beyond the data analysis team.

5.13.5 Consequence Analysis

Examining the consequences of implementing an association rule in practice can assess its potential impact and real-world implications. This step is crucial for translating insights into actionable strategies and maximizing the practical value of the discovered patterns.

5.14 Case Studies and Examples in Reproductive Medicine: Illuminating Clinical Practice

Reproductive medicine encompasses a vibrant constellation of interventions aimed at optimizing reproductive function, treating infertility, and facilitating healthy pregnancies (Djenouri et al. 2014). While statistics and research papers provide broad strokes, delving into individual case studies illuminates the intricate nuances of this field, showcasing the impact of these interventions on real lives. This paper explores the power of case studies in reproductive medicine, presenting detailed examples to illustrate the diverse applications and complex considerations within this dynamic field.

5.14.1 Case Study: 1

In many fields, including clinical treatment, data mining and knowledge discovery are also being used to analyze data looking for association rules between diseases. In a study researchers talked about the reasons why medical data must be analyzed in order to expand on medical knowledge and decision (Hui et al. 2015). The paper employed association rules and decision tree methods to answer the following question: What is the relationship between endometriosis, barrenness, and alcohol treatment? Analyzing the relationships between these conditions can shed light on where we might look to derive information and useful knowledge from medical records. The aim was to distil useful information and knowledge from medical records, which can be used as a reference for doctors in clinical treatment.

In this paper patients with barrenness and normal CA values, as well as those who are currently not pregnant but have been so in the past may be unsuitable for alcohol treatment. It is in fact found that for other patients, alcohol treatment longer than 10 min can cure the disease. But more research is needed to find the optimum duration of treatment and possible side effects. It is particularly stressed that data mining plays an important role; through the use of association rules, decision tree methods can be used to analyze medical records in order to raise standards for medical care and treatment outcomes. These two methods were used respectively to test the association relationship between endometriosis, barrenness, and alcohol treatment.

A popular method in data mining, the Apriori algorithm was used to extract related associations and potential knowledge from that dataset. The aim was to use association rules, as often used in market-basket analysis, for the discovery of associations between diseases and possible knowledge. The recorded medical data was also processed using decision tree analysis, in order to derive useful information. Using medical records and applying data mining technology, the researchers generalized characteristics of patients with endometriosis or barrenness who received alcohol treatment. The purpose was to provide a reference for physicians in their own medical practice, by looking at how the association relates between these conditions.

To determine the link between endometriosis, infertility, and alcohol treatment, researchers analyzed recorded medical associated data. The study mentions the use of huge databases for data mining, suggesting that our research data likely came from medical records and others. It was deduced that the data employed in this study came from medical records and related information concerning endometriosis, sterility, and alcohol treatment. As a result of this analysis, the results could be used as references for doctors in making medical treatment decisions.

Researchers discovered that the curative effect of treatment depended chiefly on CA exponents prior to operation and barrenness. It appeared that laparotomies made little difference to the treatment result. This study found that alcohol treatment which lasted for over 10 min was most effective. Nevertheless, the results differed from those of other studies. Those patients with normal CA exponents prior to the operation had a greater chance of improving than those who fared abnormally. In addition, the prognosis of patients without barrenness was more favorable than that for those with bareness. Association rules and decision tree analysis techniques contributed to identification of associations, making it possible for physicians to find useful knowledge from medical records.

5.14.2 Case Study: 2

Classical works on sampling techniques, statistical methods, and experimental designs are the traditional materials for researching evidence-based medicine. The techniques of data mining are less well-exploited in the medical and clinical field, but there has been growing interest in their use over recent years. Beyond the boundaries of medicine: These techniques are involved in many medical applications, such as genetic analysis, decision support systems clinical management, and clinical diagnosis. Previous studies have covered evaluating and comparing data mining strategies for medical diagnostics, how to improve clinical decision support systems, as well as the difficulties of integrating human expertise into computer-based decision support. The research is focused on assessing applications that use a clinically modified info-fuzzy network algorithm along with this author's own.

These techniques can be used to examine discrete valued clinical data gathered at fertility clinics, providing insight into the relations between various attributes as well as their role in a clinical context. With the clinically modified info-fuzzy network algorithm, the dataset can be explored using questions and hypotheses based on clinical understanding. This way of flexibly analyzing data is a strength particular to this model. The hybrid composite association rule algorithm includes both conjunctions and disjunctions. In a medical context, it permits the investigation of alternative combinations. These algorithms produce results from which complex clinical questions can be answered and patterns in medical data discovered. One strength of the clinically adjusted info-fuzzy network algorithm is its ability to derive negative associations in addition to positive and nil (neutral) associates, which can clarify many questions concerning assisted reproductive technology.

The analysis of discrete valued clinical data obtained at the Westmead Fertility Clinic uses a clinically modified info-fuzzy network (IFN) algorithm (Davis et al. 2005). In addition, it uses a modified form of the composite association rule algorithm with conjunctions and disjunctions to examine many possible combinations in a medical setting. The clinically modified IFN algorithm considers not merely the statistical significance of an attribute but also its clinical importance to a given target attribute. The improved composite association rule algorithm recursively includes all useful attributes, in addition to positive and nil associations it can also generate negative ones. They're applied to a dataset for comparison and used on two test datasets to calculate their respective accuracies. The following diagram is a one-layer CMIFN.

An algorithm called the MCAR, which successively generates a large number of rules from least complex to most complicated was found to perform slightly better (Thabtah et al. 2005). This is because it deals with clinical data obtained as discrete values at Westmead Fertility Clinic. It was also discovered that the CMIFN algorithm is capable of generating negative associations, as well as positive and nil associations. The algorithms were applied to a dataset for comparison and used on two test datasets for their accuracies. Thus, the results of the algorithms were "fuzzified" according to a range determined by what is meaningful support and confidence. These algorithms permitted the examination of how various combinations might have fared in a medical setting, affording glimpses into relationships between hours spent at work and the number and size of follicles concerning pregnancy or no pregnancy.

5.14.3 Case Study: 3

In humans, POF refers to high gonadotropin ovarian failure in females before the age of 40. The symptoms include amenorrhea and infertility. The currently available treatments for POF include hormone replacement and oocyte donation which suffer from limitations in terms of long-term efficacy or side effects. Acupuncture and moxibustion treatment has been considered beneficial in POF, but the selection of acupoints differs widely among different scholars. The research hopes to explore clinical literature on the treatment of POF with acupuncture and moxibustion so that therapy can be improved, as well as work out acupoint selection rules (Han et al. 2018). The study collected literature from various databases and studied combination formulations of acupoints and their frequency. It presents objective data for future acupoint combination models and gives helpful guidance to POF therapy.

The research pinpoints the major acupoints and several important formulas of acupressure points in treating POF with such therapy. These results provide objective evidence and information on which to build future acupoint combination models for the treatment of POF. This study found that POF treatment with acupuncture and moxibustion therapy involves regulating the conception vessel (CV) and thoroughfare vessel (TV), balancing yin-yang, and promoting menstruation solution. This acupoint identification and the combination of integrative medicine can assist practitioners in their choice of suitable points for POF treatment, which would enhance the efficacy rate for therapy with acupuncture and moxibustion. The results of the study will help to standardize acupoint selection and combination for POF treatment, making it easier to duplicate in clinical practice.

Literature selection was made according to certain standards, and the articles that met these criteria were all subjected to full-text analysis. Articles that failed to make the grade were eliminated. The literature input was rigorously standardized, including author name and unit; journal title (such as issue number, month of publication); time of publishing; the specifics of the acupuncture moxibustion therapeutic regimen. Acupoint terms come originally from the Standardization Administration of China's Nomenclature and Location of Acupuncture Points. For acupoint combination pattern analysis, TCMISS 2.0 was used. GraphPad Prism 6.0 and SPSS 22.0 were employed for frequency distribution analysis; HemI1. versions for data management and analysis, Traditional Chinese Medicine Inheritance Support System (TCMISS) 2.0, Statistical Product and Service Solutions (SPSS) 22.0, He MI I. O., GraphPad Prism6 (−) were used Based on frequency and probability of occurrence, the support degree and confidence level were calculated.

In the treatment of Premature Ovarian Failure (POF) with acupuncture and moxibustion therapy, the study found that Guanyuan (CV4) and Sanyinjiao (SP6), were its core acupoints. The study found that acupuncture and moxibustion POF treatment involves regulating the conception vessel (CV) and thoroughfare vessel (TV), striking a balance between yin and yang, promoting menstruation, activating blood. These acupoint combination rules thus proved to be a valuable reference and objective basis for future construction of an acupoint combination model in POF treatment.

These studies prove how the laws of association can change reproductive medicine to a field amidst data-driven disclosures. With this exploration finally drawing to an end, it becomes clear that knowledge combining with technology is changing not only paradigms but rather engineering a great leap into the future where reproduction itself may soon look different. Let them serve as landmarks on a journey in which the accuracy of diagnosis joins forces with caring medicine, paving the way for better mornings yet to come.

5.15 Future Directions

Reproductive health is one of the most dynamic areas in healthcare and faces challenges and opportunities that can only be addressed with innovative solutions. Among the countless advancements in medical sciences and data science, association rule mining offers a way to navigate through the complexities found in massive volumes of reproductive health datasets. This transition from conventional methods toward a data-centric perspective will enable us to gain new insights, more targeted treatments, and eventually better results for those who are dealing with issues around reproduction.

Association rule mining is a branch of data mining that looks at discovering interesting relationships or associations between variables in large datasets. It becomes powerful as a methodology in reproductive health for it unearths connections among various determinants like genes, lifestyles, choices, and environments. The potential uses of association rule mining on reproductive health are numerous given its intersection with technology. This section embarks on a journey into the future of association rule mining in the domain of reproductive health, delving into the burgeoning possibilities that lie ahead.

A study conducted provides a new basis for the clinical and basic research of traditional Chinese medicine in the treatment of uterine fibroids, but it still needs the verification of expert interpretation, experimental research, and other methods (Jianyan Xuan et al. 2020). To combine theory with practice still needs further verification of animal experiments, clinical trials, and clinical applications. Another research on Comparing Data Mining Techniques in HIV Testing Prediction suggests that interested researchers should explore the application of data mining techniques in the healthcare industry or related settings in the future (Hailu 2015).

A paper entitled "Analysing Lifestyle and Environmental Factors on Semen Fertility using Association Rule Mining" suggests that further research can be conducted to explore the impact of additional lifestyle and environmental factors on semen fertility using association rule mining (Ahmed and Anwar 2014). The use of other data mining algorithms, in addition to the Apriori algorithm, can be explored to analyze the relationship between lifestyle and environmental factors and male fertility potential.

Researchers in their study accredited as "Analysis of Clinical Medication Rule of Trigonellae Semen Based on Data Mining" recommended further exploration of the clinical medication rule of Trigonellae Semen and analysis of its potential compatibility relationship with other traditional Chinese medicines (TCM). Importance should be given to the compatibility of Trigonellae Semen with Cyperi Rhizoma, Semen Litchi, Corydalis Rhizoma, Angelica, Prepared Rhubarb, and Rhizoma Smilacis Glabrae to enhance its clinical efficacy. Expansion and extension of the clinical application of Trigonellae Semen to fully utilize its medical characteristics (Qiao et al. 2019). Identification of the potential relationship between Trigonellae Semen and other TCM through existing medication methods. Providing data reference for further in-depth study of Trigonellae Semen.

A study conducted on "Semen quality and waiting time to pregnancy explored using association mining" emphasized that further research could explore the associations between semen parameters and waiting time to pregnancy (TTP) in larger study populations to validate the findings (Romero Herrera et al. 2021). Investigate the impact of other factors, such as lifestyle and environmental factors, on TTP in combination with semen parameters. Conduct longitudinal studies to assess the long-term effects of semen parameters on TTP and fertility outcomes. Explore the use of advanced statistical techniques, such as machine learning algorithms, to better predict TTP based on combinations of semen parameters and other variables. Investigate the potential role of genetic factors in semen quality and TTP. Conduct studies to understand the underlying mechanisms behind the negative impact of female partner age on TTP and explore potential interventions to mitigate this effect.

This will help researchers and health workers to understand the intricate network of associations found in reproductive health datasets that will assist them in knowing such things as the determinants of fertility, maternal health or genetic predispositions with a view to developing targeted interventions, preventive strategies, and personalized healthcare approaches.

In this chapter, we went through association rule mining in reproductive health, highlighting its successes and challenges. We also look at cutting-edge technologies that have a potential for transformative change such as artificial intelligence (AI), machine learning (ML) and big data analytics which are poised to redefine the landscape of reproductive health research. Working together, we can untangle the complex web of relationships underlying reproductive health—where data-driven insights empower individuals, inform healthcare choices, and improve reproductive medicine overall.

References

Ahmed N, Anwar MA (2014) Analyzing lifestyle and environmental factors on semen fertility using association rule mining. https://api.semanticscholar.org/CorpusID:198719473

Bao F, Mao L, Zhu Y et al (2021) An improved evaluation methodology for mining association rules. Axioms 11:17. https://doi.org/10.3390/axioms11010017

Davis J, Illingworth P, Salam A (2005) Applications of data mining techniques in assisted reproductive technology. https://aisel.aisnet.org/acis2005/16/

Djenouri Y, Gheraibia Y, Mehdi M et al (2014) An efficient measure for evaluating association rules. In: 2014 6th international conference of Soft Computing and Pattern Recognition (SoCPaR). IEEE, Tunis, pp 406–410
Fesahat F, Montazeri F, Hoseini SM (2020) Preimplantation genetic testing in assisted reproduction technology. J Gynecol Obstet Hum Reprod 49:101723. https://doi.org/10.1016/j.jogoh.2020.101723
Hailu TG (2015) Comparing data mining techniques in HIV testing prediction. IIM 07:153–180. https://doi.org/10.4236/iim.2015.73014
Hamad GG, Curet M (2010) Minimally invasive surgery. Am J Surg 199:263–265. https://doi.org/10.1016/j.amjsurg.2009.05.008
Han X, Fan Y, Zhao H et al (2018) Acupoint selection rule mining of premature ovarian failure treatment with acupuncture and moxibustion based on the data analysis of clinical literature. In: 2018 IEEE international conference on Bioinformatics and Biomedicine (BIBM). IEEE, Madrid, pp 1866–1871
Hegland M (2007) The apriori algorithm—a tutorial. In: Lecture Notes Series, Institute for Mathematical Sciences, National University of Singapore. WORLD SCIENTIFIC, pp 209–262
Hui L, Keh H-C, Huang N-C et al (2015) A research of applying association rules and decision tree to endometriosis. In: Li X-L, Cao T, Lim E-P et al (eds) Trends and applications in knowledge discovery and data mining. Springer International Publishing, Cham, pp 113–124
Ish Nath Jha SB (2013) An analysis on association rule mining techniques. In: International conference on Computing, Communication and Sensor Network CCSN2012, pp 40–45
Kaushik M, Sharma R, Peious SA et al (2021) A systematic assessment of numerical association rule mining methods. SN Comput Sci 2:348. https://doi.org/10.1007/s42979-021-00725-2
Kerana Hanirex D, Kaliyamurthie KP (2016) Mining frequent Itemsets in association rule mining using improved SETM algorithm. In: Dash SS, Bhaskar MA, Panigrahi BK, Das S (eds) Artificial intelligence and evolutionary computations in engineering systems. Springer India, New Delhi, pp 765–773
Khurana K (2013) A comparative analysis of association rules mining algorithms. Int J Sci Res Publ 3(5) (ISSN: 2250-3153). http://www.ijsrp.org/research-paper-0513.php?rp=P171249
Kushnir VA, Smith GD, Adashi EY (2022) The future of IVF: the new Normal in human reproduction. Reprod Sci 29:849–856. https://doi.org/10.1007/s43032-021-00829-3
Muhlenbach F, Rakotomalala R (2005) Discretization for continuous attributes. In: Wang J (ed) Encyclopedia of data warehousing and mining. IGI Global, pp 397–402
Neri QV, Lee B, Rosenwaks Z et al (2014) Understanding fertilization through intracytoplasmic sperm injection (ICSI). Cell Calcium 55:24–37. https://doi.org/10.1016/j.ceca.2013.10.006
Prasad KH, Faruquie TA, Joshi S et al (2011) Data cleansing techniques for large enterprise datasets. In: 2011 annual SRII global conference. IEEE, San Jose, pp 135–144
Qiao J-Y, Chen J, Shi J-J, Miao M-S (2019) Analysis of clinical medication rule of Trigonellae Semen based on data mining. In: Proceedings of the 5th annual International Conference on Management, Economics and Social Development (ICMESD 2019). Atlantis Press, Suzhou
Romero Herrera JA, Bang AK, Priskorn L et al (2021) Semen quality and waiting time to pregnancy explored using association mining. Andrology 9:577–587. https://doi.org/10.1111/andr.12924
Smith C, Armour M, Ee C (2016) Complementary therapies and medicines and reproductive medicine. Semin Reprod Med 34:067–073. https://doi.org/10.1055/s-0035-1571194
Thabtah F, Cowling P, Peng Y (2005) MCAR: multi-class classification based on association rule. In: The 3rd ACS/IEEE international conference on computer systems and applications, 2005. IEEE, Cairo, pp 130–136
Uyar A, Bener A, Ciray HN, Bahceci M (2009) A frequency based encoding technique for transformation of categorical variables in mixed IVF dataset. In: 2009 annual international conference of the IEEE engineering in medicine and biology society. IEEE, Minneapolis, pp 6214–6217
Wan X (2019) Influence of feature scaling on convergence of gradient iterative algorithm. J Phys Conf Ser 1213:032021. https://doi.org/10.1088/1742-6596/1213/3/032021
Wang R, Pan W, Jin L et al (2019) Artificial intelligence in reproductive medicine. Reproduction 158:R139–R154. https://doi.org/10.1530/REP-18-0523

Xuan J, Deng G, Liu R et al (2020) Analysis of medication data of women with uterine fibroids based on data mining technology. J Infect Public Health 13:1513–1516. https://doi.org/10.1016/j.jiph.2019.07.017

Yazgana P, Kusakci AO (2016) A literature survey on association rule mining algorithms. Southeast Eur J Soft Comput 5. https://doi.org/10.21533/scjournal.v5i1.102

Yedjour D, Benyettou A (2018) Symbolic interpretation of artificial neural networks based on multiobjective genetic algorithms and association rules mining. Appl Soft Comput 72:177–188. https://doi.org/10.1016/j.asoc.2018.08.007

Yuan X (2017) An improved Apriori algorithm for mining association rules. AIP Conf Proc 1820:080005

Zhang W, Liao H, Zhao N (2008) Research on the FP growth algorithm about association rule mining. In: 2008 international seminar on business and information management. IEEE, Wuhan, pp 315–318

Zhao Q, Bhowmick S (2003) Association rule mining: a survey. In: Technical report, CAIS, nanyang technological university, Singapore. https://personal.ntu.edu.sg/assourav/Unpublished/UP-ARMSurvey.pdf. Accessed 1 Oct 2024

Modeling in Reproductive Health and Treatment Outcomes

6

Sudipta Sardar, Somenath Dutta, and Ganesh Jadhav

Abstract

This chapter explores the pivotal role of Support Vector Regression (SVR) as a machine-learning technique in bioinformatics. It outlines the mathematical foundations of SVR, including kernel functions and hyperparameters. A key advantage of SVR is its ability to model complex biological relationships by fitting nonlinear data in high-dimensional space. Through real-world examples, the chapter demonstrates SVR's efficacy across diverse bioinformatics applications, unlocking novel insights. Additionally, the chapter emphasizes SVR's immense potential to enable breakthroughs in life sciences research and data analysis, also highlighting the associated limitations. Building on the success of Support Vector Machines (SVM) in classification, the chapter introduces Support Vector Regression (SVR) for regression tasks, and how SVR balances model complexity and error tolerance by minimizing error within a tube. Furthermore, we showcase an example application of leveraging SVR to create a virtual screening prediction tool that highlights its strength in handling both linear and nonlinear regression problems. Overall, the chapter serves as a valuable guide to SVR, emphasizing its capacity to yield profound insights from biological data.

S. Sardar
Department of Bioinformatics, Pondicherry Central University, Puducherry, India

S. Dutta (✉)
Department of Bioinformatics, Pondicherry Central University, Puducherry, India

IHub-Data, International Institute of Information Technology, Hyderabad, India
e-mail: somenath@bicpu.edu.in

G. Jadhav
IHub-Data, International Institute of Information Technology, Hyderabad, India

A. Sengupta et al. (eds.), *Data-Driven Reproductive Health*,
https://doi.org/10.1007/978-981-97-7451-7_6

Keywords

Machine learning · SVR · SVM · CADD · Virtual screening · Male fertility

6.1 Introduction

Machine Learning (ML) serves as a pivotal branch in computer science that enables computers to *"learn"* from the provided data. In this context, learning refers to the identification of hidden patterns within the input data empowering the machine to predict future unseen data points based on prior knowledge. Several machine learning algorithms are available, and they differ in their principal mathematical computation to discern the underlying pattern (Learning). Machine learning can be categorized into two main subtypes—Supervised learning and Unsupervised learning.

Supervised learning is a type of machine learning where the model is trained on a labeled dataset, which means the input data is paired with the corresponding correct output in the dataset. The goal of supervised learning algorithms is to find the underlying pattern that can efficiently map between the input and the output and then make predictions for the unseen input data. Some well-known supervised machine learning algorithms include *Random Forest (RF)*, Decision Tree, *Support Vector Machine (SVM), K-Nearest Neighbors (KNN)*, and more. Conversely, unsupervised learning, on the other hand, involves training algorithms on unlabeled data where the algorithm is not provided with explicit output labels. The goal of unsupervised learning is to find the pattern or relationship within the data without guidance of what the output should be. While supervised learning has extensive applications in classification and regression tasks, unsupervised learning is commonly used for tasks like clustering and dimensionality reduction. Commonly used unsupervised machine learning algorithms include Principal Component Analysis (PCA), K-means clustering, and more (Sarker 2021).

6.2 Support Vector Machine (SVM)

Support Vector Machine (SVM) stands out as one of the most popular and efficient supervised machine learning algorithms capable of adeptly handling both classification and regression tasks. In the realm of bioinformatics, where the classification and prediction of biological data are pivotal, the utilization of computer programs for automating the classification process has become indispensable. This is especially crucial as biological data banks continue to witness a rapid surge in size. Despite its prevalence in solving classification problems, the application of SVM in regression remains relatively uncommon. Nevertheless, SVMs have earned extensive recognition and use within the field of bioinformatics (Yang 2004). They have proven successful in a variety of applications, including protein structure prediction (Zangooei and Jalili 2012; Qiu et al. 2008), protein-protein binding affinity

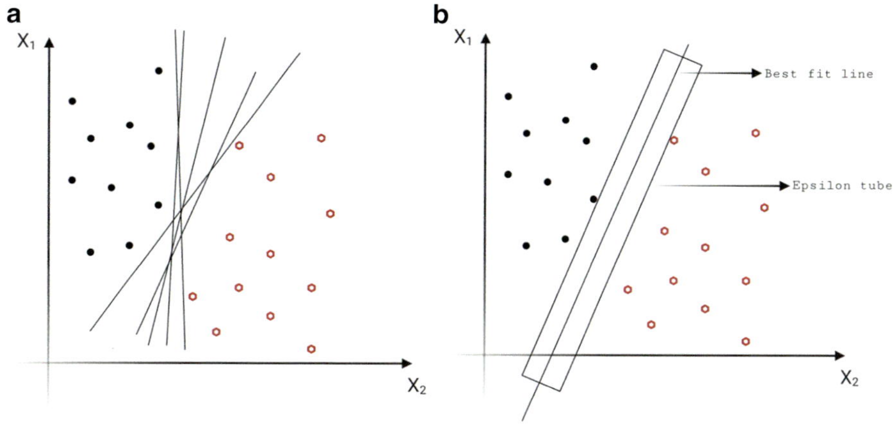

Fig. 6.1 Understanding optimal hyperplane (**a**) multiple hyperplanes (lines in black) can be drawn to separate two distinct classes (marked in red and black); (**b**) the optimal hyperplane should have an equal distance on both sides while considering the maximum margin from both classes

prediction (Liu et al. 2006), protein solvent accessibility prediction (Wagner et al. 2005), gene expression data analysis, and more (Brown et al. 2000). The distinguishing factor that contributes to SVM's efficacy lies in its algorithm's focus on maximizing the margin between two classes. This contrasts with other algorithms that primarily aim to minimize the errors during the training process, often resulting in poorer generalization. With a given dataset, SVM tries to find a line that can differentiate between two lines, referred to as a "hyperplane", as depicted in Fig. 6.1a. In a two-dimensional space, a hyperplane is simply a straight line. However, when dealing with more than two features in higher-dimensional space, the hyperplane transforms into a flat sub-space.

SVM seeks to identify the optimal hyperplane (often termed "the best-fit line") as illustrated in Fig. 6.1b within an *N*-dimensional space, characterized by the maximum margin from the closest data points in each class, commonly known as Support Vectors (Boser et al. 1992). While the fundamental principle remains constant, SVM can handle both linear and nonlinear problem types, classifying the SVM into *Linear SVMs (LSVMs)* and *Nonlinear SVMs*. However, in the realm of SVMs, distinct methodologies have emerged to cater to specific tasks: *Support Vector Classification (SVC)* for classification purposes and *Support Vector Regression (SVR)* to address regression challenges (Stafford Noble 2006; Byvatov and Schneider 2003).

6.3 Support Vector Regression (SVR)

Support Vector Regression (SVR), as a type of SVM, follows the same fundamental principles with nuanced distinctions. When presented with data points, SVR endeavors to identify a hyperplane. Unlike its classification counterpart, SVR, being a

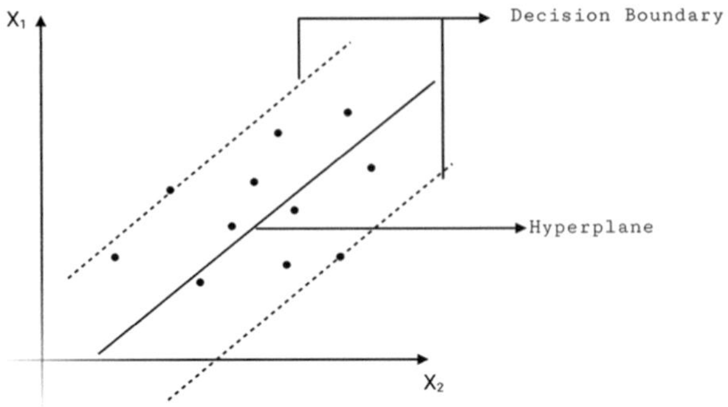

Fig. 6.2 Support vector regression (SVR) includes maximum data points inside decision boundaries (ε-tube) and the hyperplane maintains an equal distance from both decision boundaries

regression algorithm, does not employ the hyperplane as a decision boundary; instead, it utilizes the curve to establish a correlation between the vector and the curve's position. Support Vectors play a crucial role in discerning the closest match between the data points and the corresponding function representing them in Fig. 6.2.

In most traditional regression models, the primary objective is to minimize the *Root Mean Squared Error (RMSE)*. However, SVR introduces a unique concept by adding flexibility to the model, allowing it to tolerate errors up to a certain threshold. While the overarching goal remains to minimize errors, SVR is founded on the idea of finding the optimal value within a margin threshold known as epsilon tube (tube of tolerance or margin of tolerance). This approach considers the necessity to minimize errors for a given set of input variables.

In the realm of regression, SVR demonstrates versatility by adeptly handling both linear and nonlinear tasks. Within SVR, regression unfolds in a higher-dimensional feature space achieved through the transformation of input data using a kernel function. This kernel, in turn, dictates the shape of the decision boundary based on the best-fit curve, enabling SVR to navigate nonlinear relationships between input variables and target variables within an optimal hyperplane. The kernel, essentially a set of mathematical functions, maps data points into higher-dimensional space and transforms them as needed. There are several common kernel functions available such as Polynomial, Linear, Sigmoid, *Radial Basis Function (RBF)*. This mechanism empowers the SVR model to implicitly function in a higher-dimensional space without the explicit computation of transformed features.

In the domain of bioinformatics, *Support Vector Regression (SVR)* plays a pivotal role. Its application extends to various areas such as the study of bioactivities of chemical compounds, prediction of antioxidant activity of phenolic compounds, prediction of protein secondary structure, and more (Shi 2021; Zangooei and Jalili 2012; Zhou et al. 2006).

The adaptability of SVR in handling nonlinear relationships makes it a valuable tool in bioinformatics research, especially where traditional regression models may fall short of capturing the complexity of biological data (Sethi 2024).

6.3.1 Hyperparameter Optimization

Hyperparameters are a set of instructions or parameters, whose values control the learning process and determine parameter values that a learning algorithm ends up learning with, they serve as crucial instructions set by data scientists based on prior domain knowledge, experience, or through a process of trial and error. The prefix "hyper" means they are "top-level" and that they control the learning process. These configurations are external and have to be defined before model training as these cannot be learned from the training data. In SVR, several hyperparameters play pivotal roles as discussed below.

6.3.1.1 Epsilon

It defines the width of the epsilon tube around the hyperplane, which is the decision boundary that separates the data points in n-dimensional space. However, a smaller epsilon value is suitable for tasks where capturing fine details is necessary but may overfit the training data and a higher epsilon value may be more appropriate for noisy data, where some extents of errors are acceptable. So, the choice of epsilon value significantly impacts the performance of the SVR model.

6.3.1.2 Kernel

Selecting an appropriate kernel is crucial for complex datasets, where the dataset is not separable linearly. By default, the SVR takes the linear kernel, but we can explicitly mention the kernel function using this parameter. Usually, computational cost increases if we increase the dimension of the data. A kernel function helps us to find a hyperplane in higher-dimensional space without increasing the computational cost.

6.3.1.3 Gamma

This parameter controls the width of the *Radial Basis Function (RBF)* kernel. RBF is a commonly used kernel in SVR. A higher value of gamma leads to a narrower kernel decision boundary, while a smaller gamma value results in a wider decision boundary of the kernel.

6.3.1.4 Cost Parameter

To comprehend how SVR minimizes errors within the epsilon tube while considering the trade-off between the model complexity and error tolerance, the Cost Parameter comes into play. A higher C value leads to a more complex model with a smaller margin, but it is also more prone to overfitting. Conversely, a lower C value results in a simpler model with a larger margin, but it may not capture the underlying structure in the data effectively.

The process of selecting optimal values for these hyperparameters is known as Hyperparameter Optimization. The selection of optimal values during the training step is crucial and has important implications for the model performance. Finding the optimal values can be done in various ways like grid search, random selection, or Bayesian optimization.

6.3.2 Mathematical Underpinnings of SVR

SVR relies on intricate mathematical algorithms and optimization techniques that underpin its performance. To fully understand the effectiveness of SVR, it is required to delve into the mathematical insights. Before diving into the underpinnings of SVR we have to know some fundamentals of *Support Vector Classifier (SVC)*. In this case, we will be understanding the simplest SVM, which is *LSVM*.

6.3.2.1 Data Points, Support Vectors, and Epsilon Tube

Suppose we have a dataset as shown in Table 6.1, where we have feature matrix X and corresponding class Y. The first task is to find the best-fit line using support vectors.

As demonstrated in Fig. 6.3a, any of the drawn lines can correctly separate two classes. This line is called a hyperplane. But if we take a hyperplane that is close to "Class 1" the model can be biased towards "Class 1" and vice versa. So, which one will be the best-fit line? To find the best-fit line we use the idea of maximum margin. The marginal plane would be increased until it touches the marginal data points (Support Vectors) on both sides. The width of the margin will be the same on both sides, as illustrated in Fig. 6.3b.

As shown in Fig. 6.3c the distance between the hyperplane and the marginal plane will be ε on each side. So, the total margin will be:

$$m = 2\varepsilon$$

which is also the width of the epsilon tube.

Now the equation of the hyperplane can be represented as

$$W^T X + b = 0$$

where

W = Normal vector
X = Input vector
b = Bias

and the marginal planes can be represented as

$$W^T X + b = +1,$$
$$\text{and} \qquad W^T X + b = -1$$

Table 6.1 Example dataset

X_1	X_2	X_3		Y
a_1	b_1	c_1	...	Class 1
a_2	b_2	c_2	...	Class 2
...	....	...	...	...
a_n	b_n	c_n	...	Class 1

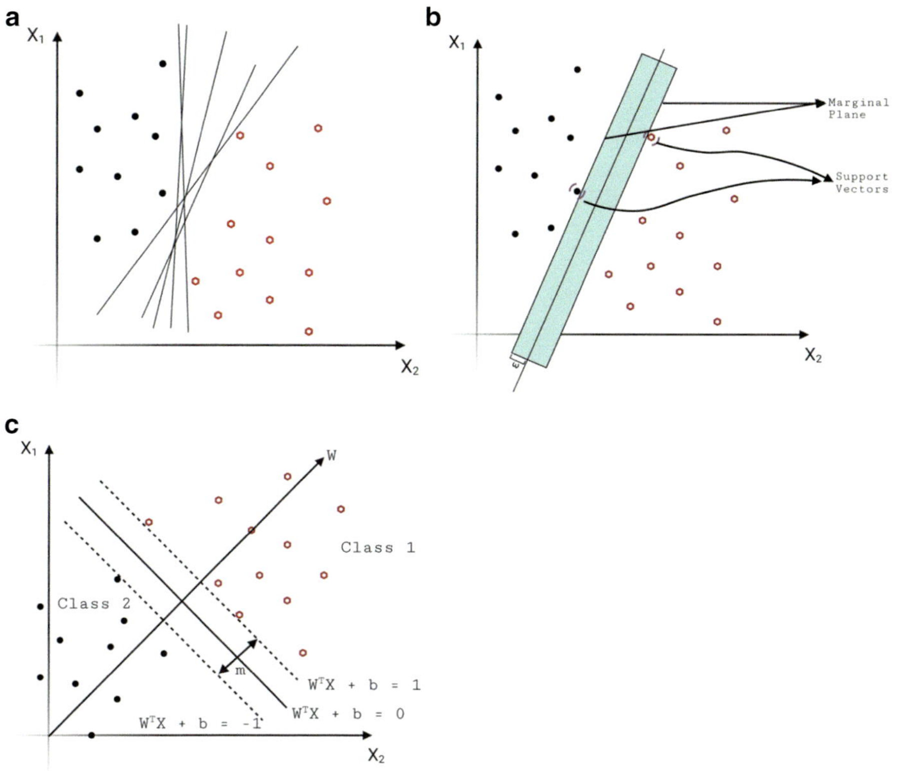

Fig. 6.3 Support vector machine **(a)** multiple hyperplanes can be drawn to separate two distinct classes; **(b)** hyperplane with maximum margin from both decision boundaries (support vectors) will be considered as best-fit line forming a tube-like structure called epsilon tube; **(c)** mathematical underpinnings of SVM

6.3.2.1.1 Discriminant Function

Now, the discriminant function is:

$$y_i = W^T X + b$$

with aim,
for each correct classification

$$W^T X + b \geq +1 \text{ for "Class 1"}$$
$$\text{and } W^T X + b \leq -1 \text{ for "Class 2"}$$

Now, for all data points, we can multiply the above two equations:

$$y_i \left(W^T X + b \right) \geq +1$$

6.3.2.1.2 Objective Function

We aim to maximize the margin m. The distance between two marginal planes will be

$$W^T X_1 + b = +1\ldots \quad (6.1)$$

$$W^T X_2 + b = -1\ldots \quad (6.2)$$

After subtracting Eq. (6.1) and Eq. (6.2), we get

$$W^T (X_1 - X_2) = 2$$

$$\text{or} \quad \frac{W^T}{\|W\|}(X_1 - X_2) = \frac{2}{\|W\|}$$

$$\text{or} \quad \text{margin}(m) = \frac{2}{\|W\|}$$

So, our objective function will be

$$\textit{maximize}\ \text{margin}(m) = \textit{minimize}\|W\|$$

with constraints $y_i(W^T X + b) \geq +1$ for data points.

6.3.2.2 SVR and Its Errors

So, enough fundamentals of SVM, but the SVR, as it is used for regression problems, tries to find the best-fit curve while positioning maximum data points inside the epsilon tube as shown in Fig. 6.4. For each correctly fitted data points the constraints in SVR will be

$$y_i - W^T X \leq \varepsilon$$

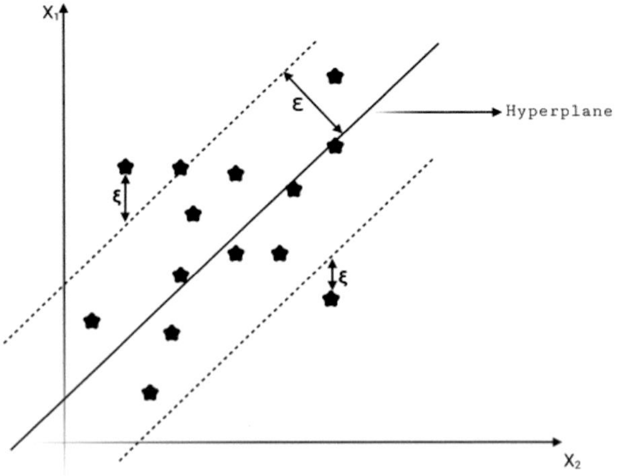

Fig. 6.4 Errors in SVR: distance of data points from the decision boundaries will be considered as error

In real-world scenarios, especially the biological datasets are noisy. But what if we allow some level of errors during training? This can be done with the cost parameter C and error ξ. So, the loss function will be

$$\text{Loss function} = \frac{1}{2}\|W\| + C\sum_{i=1}^{n}\xi_i$$

where C = number of data points that can be outside of the epsilon tube
ξ = distance from the marginal plane

C is a hyperparameter, where it trades off the relative importance of maximizing the margin and fitting the training data. The error is calculated by measuring the distance between the marginal plane and the data point outside the epsilon tube. So, the final constraints of the SVR will be

$$y_i - W^T X \leq \varepsilon + \xi_i$$

6.4 Advantages of SVR

Key advantages of using *Support Vector Regression (SVR)* include, but are not limited to the following.

6.4.1 Complex Modeling

Biological systems are often characterized by intricate nonlinear relationships. SVR can capture these complex nonlinear relationships in data using kernel tricks, making it well-suited for biological systems. This makes SVR even better than neural networks.

6.4.2 Data Overfitting

The appropriate selection of epsilon value controls the width of the epsilon tube, which eventually enhances the capability of generalization, reducing the data overfitting.

6.4.3 Robustness

One of the main problems in bioinformatics is that biological data are often noisy due to experimental errors. However, SVR's ε-insensitive loss function makes it suitable for noisy biological datasets less susceptible to outliers.

6.5 Disadvantages of SVR

Despite its numerous advantages, SVR has some drawbacks also.

6.5.1 Computational Cost

SVR has complex mathematical algorithms underlying, making it computationally expensive during training time, especially for large datasets and complex kernel functions. This can be a limiting factor for individual researchers where computational resources are limited.

6.5.2 Choice of Kernel

The kernel function has heavy implications for the performance of the model. Selecting an appropriate kernel for a particular dataset is a crucial task and needs subject matter expertise, making it difficult for beginner bioinformaticians.

6.5.3 Hyperparameter Tuning

Selecting optimal hyperparameters of the kernel requires careful experimentation and may be time-consuming.

However, despite its limitations, SVR gave promising results in balancing the accuracy and predictability in the field of modern-day bioinformatics. To bridge the gap between the theory and practice, here we include an example showcasing the efficiency of SVR in bioinformatics.

6.6 SVR in Action: A Virtual Screening Prediction Tool

In the realm of drug discovery, computational methodologies play a crucial role in hastening the identification of potential drug candidates. This involves pinpointing specific receptors, such as proteins or RNA, and delving into their interactions with diverse ligands and chemical molecules with the potential to act as therapeutic agents. A key strategy in this endeavor is virtual screening, a computational technique meticulously crafted to efficiently sift through extensive ligand libraries, pinpointing those most likely to bind effectively to a designated target receptor. Instead of physically testing thousands or millions of compounds in a laboratory, virtual screening uses computer algorithms and simulations to prioritize and filter potential drug candidates.

The rapid progress in machine learning within the specialized domain has captured the attention of researchers in drug discovery and computational chemistry. Numerous studies have underscored the promising outcomes of employing virtual screening prediction tools that leverage machine learning and structure-based descriptors. To exemplify this procedure, we will delve into a practical case study, offering a detailed examination outlined in Fig. 6.5, showcasing the creation of a

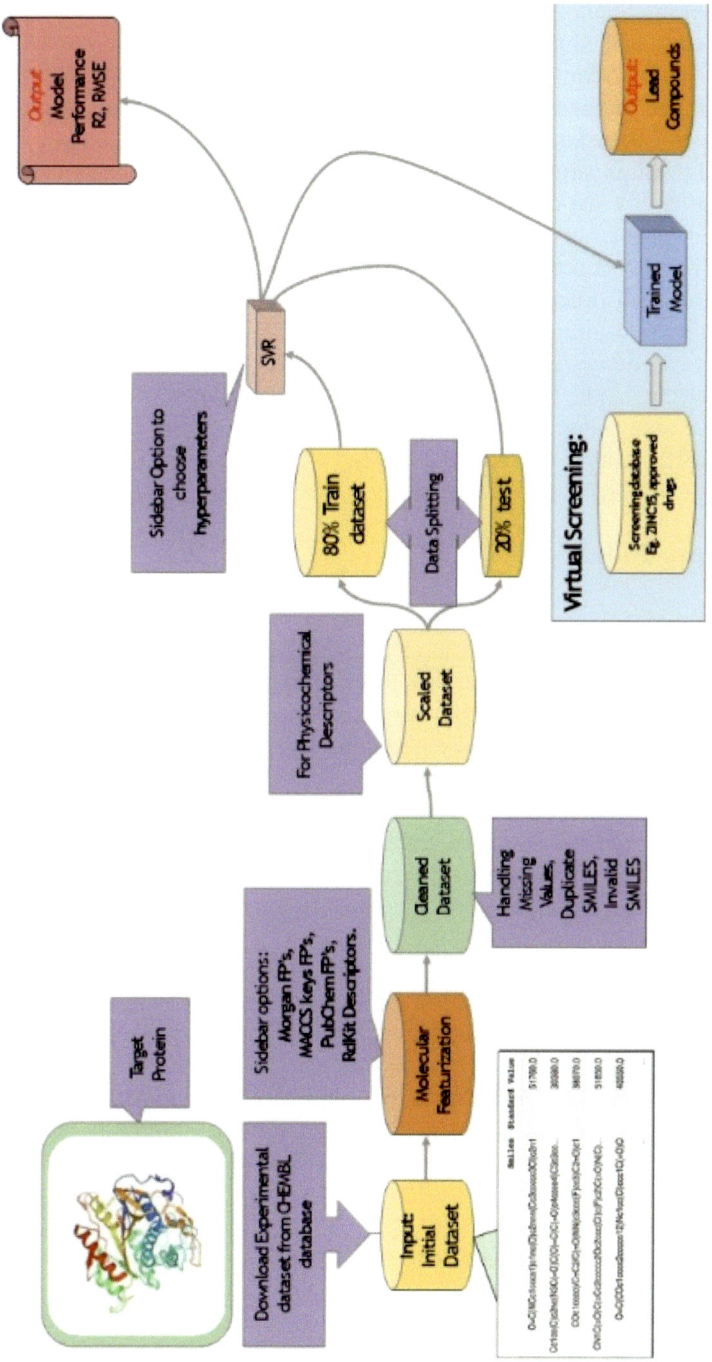

Fig. 6.5 Schematic representation of the virtual screening tool development process

customized virtual screening tool aimed at uncovering inhibitors of Aromatase, a highly intriguing field of study.

Aromatase, an enzyme crucial in estrogen biosynthesis from androgens, converts androgens like testosterone into estrogens, predominantly estradiol. It is present in multiple tissues including ovaries, testes, and brain. In males, it maintains the androgen-estrogen balance essential for normal reproductive function. Targeting aromatase is vital in several medical contexts. Aromatase inhibitors treat hormone receptor-positive breast cancer by reducing estrogen production. In male infertility cases, excess aromatase activity is corrected to restore hormone balance and potentially enhance sperm production. These inhibitors also regulate hormone levels in estrogen-related disorders and facilitate drug development through research into aromatase's role, offering new treatment avenues. Essentially, targeting aromatase is crucial for hormone regulation, hormone-related cancer treatment, male infertility management, and progress in drug research and development. Through this example, we aim to demonstrate practical insights into the creation of such a tool (Schlegel 2012; Raman and Schlegel 2002).

6.6.1 Data Collection

The first step of any machine learning problem requires sufficient experimentally validated data to build a reliable model. ChEMBL is an open access resource of compound structures and their biological activities, primarily abstracted and curated from scientific literature. ChEMBL web resource client suite can be used to download data using python seamlessly (Gaulton et al. 2017). In our case assay data containing compounds targeting Aromatase was downloaded from the ChEMBL database using the chembl_webresource_client suite (Davies et al. 2015). The molecules in the dataset were represented by *SMILES (Simple Molecular-Input Line-Entry System)* along with other assay information. In the dataset, columns contained molecular structure and their IC50 values are our area of interest to build the virtual screening tool (Zhou et al. 2021).

First, we **collect data** on small molecules, represented using SMILES strings alongside their corresponding activity values. These SMILES are then **featurized** to generate a suitable dataset. Subsequently, the data undergoes a **cleaning process** to eliminate redundancies and address missing entries. To optimize the model's efficiency, **feature selection techniques** are employed for dimensionality reduction. Finally, the dataset is **split** in an 80:20 ratio for training and testing purposes. The trained model's performance is further **validated** using an external dataset.

6.6.2 Molecular Featurization

To enable machine learning modeling, the molecular structures in the dataset first required transformation into structured descriptive inputs from its SMILE format. Recent research has demonstrated that predictive models built using structure-based descriptors can achieve accuracy rivaling approaches relying on intensive quantum calculations (Sandfort et al. 2020). There are several structure-based descriptors such as Morgan FPs, PubChem FPs, MACCs Key FPs, and more. RDKit, a chemoinformatics and machine learning software written in Python, was used for calculating molecular descriptors such as molecular weight, LogP, number of hydrogen acceptors, and number of hydrogen donors of molecule from SMILES notation (Landrum et al. 2024). For the simplicity of this showcasing example, we calculated only a set of PubChem fingerprints and molecular descriptors using PADEL-Descriptor software (Yap 2011). This takes SMILES as input and returns set of descriptors and fingerprints model for virtual screening of new Aromatase inhibitors.

6.6.3 Dataset Cleaning & Preparation

After calculating molecular descriptors, the dataset was left with molecular descriptors and their corresponding pIC50 values and required significant preprocessing and cleaning before it could be used for the model training. Duplicate structures that may have different assay results were removed since duplicate entries would affect the performance of the model. Also, entries with missing IC50 and SMILES values were eliminated from the dataset. IC50 values are then converted into pIC50 values to normalize the data using the below equation, which is a widespread practice in drug discovery (Selvaraj et al. 2011).

$$pIC_{50} = -\log_{10}\left(IC_{50}\right)$$

Following this, Lipinski's rule of five (RO5) descriptors were calculated for each molecule from its SMILES notation using RDKit python package. Lipinski's RO5 is a thumb rule to evaluate if a chemical compound would be orally active drug in humans and describes molecular properties important for drug's pharmacokinetics, including their *ADME (Absorption, Distribution, Metabolism, and Excretion)* properties. The descriptors include molecular weight, hydrogen bond donors, hydrogen bond acceptors, and *octanol-water partition coefficient (ClogP)*. Compounds violating more than one of the Lipinski criteria were removed as they are likely to have poor oral absorption and permeability.

6.6.4 Scaled Dataset

After rigorous data preprocessing steps, the dataset needs to be scaled down as the dimensionality of molecular descriptors are high and might affect the model performance by overfitting. Thus, to select relevant features, dimensionality reduction techniques like *PCA* and *t-Distributed Stochastic Neighbor Embedding (t-SNE)* techniques could be applied. However, we have adopted feature selection techniques like Variance Threshold and Pearson Correlation Matrix to reduce the dimensionality embedded in the Scikit-learn library. The Variance Threshold method facilitates the identification of features with low variance, which may contribute to overfitting. We can refine the dataset by removing columns with constant values by selecting a threshold, in this case, zero. By ensuring that only informative characteristics are kept, this procedure improves the discriminative capability of the model. In order to prevent redundancy and potential overfitting, we simultaneously use the Pearson Correlation Matrix to evaluate the correlation coefficient between each pair of features. This analysis allows us to identify highly correlated features, as a correlation coefficient closer to ±1 indicates stronger associations. To prevent redundancy and potential overfitting, we discard features with a correlation coefficient greater than or equal to 80%. The remaining dataset, free from highly correlated features, serves as the foundation for model training. It is noteworthy that, in addition to the aforementioned techniques, alternative feature selection methods could be explored to further address overfitting concerns.

6.6.5 Model Construction

Now the scaled-down molecular descriptors can better capture relevant properties and enable the model robust by avoiding overfitting. Scikit-learn is a free machine learning library for Python, which includes various machine learning algorithms for classification, regression, and clustering. Using the scikit-learn SVR and RF, models were trained under the Google Collaboratory environment in our case. The dataset is first randomly separated into an 80:20 training and test set ratio. Based on the training data and specified algorithms used, a specified set of hyperparameters was optimized with a fivefold cross-validation strategy to find out the combination that achieved minimum loss. Grid Search strategy was used to find these optimal hyperparameter values. The model's performance on the training set was evaluated for each combination of hyperparameter values and the final model was constructed based on these assessments.

6.6.6 Model Performance

Now, the model's predictive performance was assessed on a "holdout" test set using the coefficient of determination (R2) and *root-mean-squared error (RMSE)*, and the best-performing, fine-tuned algorithm on the test set was deployed for virtual screening based on its high R2 and low RMSE.

6.6.7 Model Deployment and Virtual Screening

After the successful development of the model, the model file was dumped as a pickle object, and streamlit library was used to build an interactive web application. This web interface gives options to select a particular set of descriptors for the model. Now we can input a CSV file, containing SMILES of molecules and the web application will convert SMILES into the selected set of feature descriptors internally.

Then the model will predict the pIC50 values and return results in the web interface. A pIC50 value of 7 or more is considered a potent inhibitor of Aromatase.

A deployed version of the model in a web application can be accessed at https://fertility.streamlit.app/ and the source code is provided at https://github.com/49357514/VS-app for the reference to build such models.

6.7 Conclusion

While SVR comes with its limitations in terms of computational expenses, choice of kernels, and tedious optimization of hyperparameters, it provides state-of-the-art capabilities in modeling noisy biological data. Its mathematical sophistication empowers it to capture intricate nonlinear relationships and complex high-dimensional patterns prevalent in biological systems. Underpinned by concepts of margin maximization rather than pure error minimization, SVR offers enhanced generalization capabilities. The kernel trick allows SVR models to tackle nonlinear tasks through implicit mapping to higher-dimensional feature spaces. Careful hyperparameter tuning and kernel selection enable the balancing of model complexity and overfitting risks. As highlighted through the provided case study, SVR can drive innovations in bioinformatics applications ranging from protein function prediction to demonstrably effective virtual screening tools to expedite drug discovery. With its robustness against outliers and focus on maximizing margin width, SVR has rightfully claimed its place among the most widely adopted machine learning techniques within bioinformatics.

In conclusion, as both biological data and computational capabilities continue their exponential growth trajectories, SVM and SVR will only increase in utility and adoption. This book chapter has endeavored to provide readers with a comprehensive yet accessible exploration into workings, advantages, limitations, and real-world application of support vector machine in bioinformatics.

Acknowledgments The authors are incredibly thankful to the International Institute of Information Technology (IIIT), Hyderabad, and the Department of Bioinformatics, Pondicherry Central University, for rendering accession to their support in the completion of our study.

References

Boser BE, Guyon IM, Vapnik VN (1992) A training algorithm for optimal margin classifiers. In: Proceedings of the fifth annual workshop on computational learning theory. ACM, Pittsburgh, pp 144–152

Brown MPS, Grundy WN, Lin D et al (2000) Knowledge-based analysis of microarray gene expression data by using support vector machines. Proc Natl Acad Sci USA 97:262–267. https://doi.org/10.1073/pnas.97.1.262

Byvatov E, Schneider G (2003) Support vector machine applications in bioinformatics. Appl Bioinforma 2:67–77

Davies M, Nowotka M, Papadatos G et al (2015) ChEMBL web services: streamlining access to drug discovery data and utilities. Nucleic Acids Res 43:W612–W620. https://doi.org/10.1093/nar/gkv352

Gaulton A, Hersey A, Nowotka M et al (2017) The ChEMBL database in 2017. Nucleic Acids Res 45:D945–D954. https://doi.org/10.1093/nar/gkw1074

Landrum G, Tosco P, Kelley B et al (2024) rdkit/rdkit: 2023_09_6 (Q3 2023) release

Liu W, Meng X, Xu Q et al (2006) Quantitative prediction of mouse class I MHC peptide binding affinity using support vector machine regression (SVR) models. BMC Bioinformatics 7:182. https://doi.org/10.1186/1471-2105-7-182

Qiu J, Sheffler W, Baker D, Noble WS (2008) Ranking predicted protein structures with support vector regression. Proteins 71:1175–1182. https://doi.org/10.1002/prot.21809

Raman JD, Schlegel PN (2002) Aromatase inhibitors for male infertility. J Urol 167:624–629. https://doi.org/10.1016/S0022-5347(01)69099-2

Sandfort F, Strieth-Kalthoff F, Kühnemund M et al (2020) A structure-based platform for predicting chemical reactivity. Chem 6:1379–1390. https://doi.org/10.1016/j.chempr.2020.02.017

Sarker IH (2021) Machine learning: algorithms, real-world applications and research directions. SN Comput Sci 2:160. https://doi.org/10.1007/s42979-021-00592-x

Schlegel PN (2012) Aromatase inhibitors for male infertility. Fertil Steril 98:1359–1362. https://doi.org/10.1016/j.fertnstert.2012.10.023

Selvaraj C, Tripathi S, Reddy K, Singh SK (2011) Tool development for prediction of pIC50 values from the IC50 values-A pIC50 value calculator. Curr Trends Biotechnol Pharm 5:1104–1109

Sethi A (2024) Support vector regression tutorial for machine learning. In: Analytics Vidhya. https://www.analyticsvidhya.com/blog/2020/03/support-vector-regression-tutorial-for-machine-learning/

Shi Y (2021) Support vector regression-based QSAR models for prediction of antioxidant activity of phenolic compounds. Sci Rep 11:8806. https://doi.org/10.1038/s41598-021-88341-1

Stafford Noble W (2006) A biologist's introduction to support vector machines. In: Semantic Scholar. https://api.semanticscholar.org/CorpusID:7675828

Wagner M, Adamczak R, Porollo A, Meller J (2005) Linear regression models for solvent accessibility prediction in proteins. J Comput Biol 12:355–369. https://doi.org/10.1089/cmb.2005.12.355

Yang ZR (2004) Biological applications of support vector machines. Brief Bioinform 5:328–338. https://doi.org/10.1093/bib/5.4.328

Yap CW (2011) PaDEL-descriptor: An open source software to calculate molecular descriptors and fingerprints Abstract. J Comput Chem 32(7);1466–1474. https://doi.org/10.1002/jcc.v32.7

Zangooei MH, Jalili S (2012) Protein secondary structure prediction using DWKF based on SVR-NSGAII. Neurocomputing 94:87–101. https://doi.org/10.1016/j.neucom.2012.04.015

Zhou Y-P, Jiang J-H, Lin W-Q et al (2006) Boosting support vector regression in QSAR studies of bioactivities of chemical compounds. Eur J Pharm Sci 28:344–353. https://doi.org/10.1016/j.ejps.2006.04.002

Zhou J, Wu S, Lee BG et al (2021) Machine-learning-enabled virtual screening for inhibitors of lysine-specific histone demethylase 1. Molecules 26:7492. https://doi.org/10.3390/molecules26247492

Clustering Analysis of Reproductive Health Data

7

Ankita Bhatia, Jyoti Mehta, and Tarun Pal

Abstract

Reproductive health involves several phases such as fertility, menstrual cycles, and hormonal dynamics. Data-driven methodologies, like clustering analysis, help understand these complexities. This chapter discusses the different clustering algorithms that can be used on reproductive health data such as k-means, hierarchical, density-based clustering (e.g., DBSCAN), and model-based clustering (e.g., Gaussian mixture models). Furthermore, the chapter describes the preprocessing steps required to prepare reproductive data for clustering analysis focusing on the different techniques for feature selection, dimensionality reduction, and data transformation to enhance the quality and effectiveness of clustering results. It further discusses the importance of performance evaluation that could be computed using evaluation metrics which is an important determinant of the clustering algorithm's efficiency. The text describes the techniques for evaluating clusters' compactness, separation, and stability. In the last section of the chapter, various applications of clustering analysis are discussed with an interpretation of the application of clustering analysis in reproductive health.

Keywords

Reproductive health · Clustering analysis · Data exploration · Health patterns Data-driven discovery

---

A. Bhatia · J. Mehta
Faculty of Applied Sciences and Biotechnology, Shoolini University of Biotechnology and Management Sciences, Solan, Himachal Pradesh, India

T. Pal (✉)
School of Bioengineering and Food Technology, Faculty of Applied Sciences and Biotechnology, Shoolini University of Biotechnology and Management Sciences, Solan, Himachal Pradesh, India

A. Sengupta et al. (eds.), *Data-Driven Reproductive Health*,
https://doi.org/10.1007/978-981-97-7451-7_7

7.1 Introduction

Reproductive health is a complex field involving fertility, menstrual cycles, and hormonal dynamics. Data-driven methodologies, like clustering analysis, help understand these complexities. The first 6 weeks post-childbirth are crucial for survival. High-quality care is essential for the mother and baby's well-being. Improving the well-being of mothers and their babies and minimizing the negative effects of pregnancy, labor, and delivery depend on providing high-quality prenatal, intrapartum, and postnatal care. Interventions include promoting healthy diets, managing conditions, providing respectful care, supporting GBV victims, and offering mental health services (WHO 2017). Globally, 60–80 million couples experience infertility, with unsafe abortion practices causing 115,000–204,000 fatalities. Female genital mutilation persists in 40 countries. Sexually transmitted illnesses are prevalent, with adolescents, low-educated individuals, and rural dwellers at risk. It is predicted that there will be roughly 40 million HIV infections in men, women, and children shortly. A comprehensive prevention approach is needed (Rada 2014).

A worldwide perspective on reproductive health highlights the main issues that need to be addressed. The role of individuals and organizations in safeguarding reproductive health is discussed under the below categories.

7.2 Clustering Algorithms Commonly Used on Reproductive Health Data

Cluster analysis organizes data based on specific structures. Object categorization involves recognizing groupings of items that share certain qualities but differ significantly from others (Milewska et al. 2013). The clustering algorithms can be of different types such as k-means clustering, hierarchical clustering, density-based clustering (e.g., DBSCAN), and model-based clustering (e.g., Gaussian mixture models).

7.2.1 Hierarchical Algorithm

Hierarchical approaches, such as agglomerative and divisive operations, involve clustering objects into separate parts. The agglomerative method is known as a "bottom-up" strategy. Initially, each object is a separate cluster, and new clusters are produced by joining nearby objects and previously linked groups. The top-down strategy, also known as the divisive method, involves gradually breaking clustered content into single parts, unlike the previously mentioned bottom-up method. Agglomerative analytics, a bottom-up strategy, creates new clusters by joining nearby objects, while divisive methods break clustered content into single parts (Milewska et al. 2013).

The study by Dapas et al. (2020) used a clustered hierarchical approach to identify phenotypic sub-types of PCOS, validated them in an independent cohort, and determined their association with common genetic variants, and evaluated their relationship with rare genetic variation.

7.2.2 k-Means Algorithm

The k-means approach divides objects into distinct clusters without subgroups, requiring a statistician to calculate the number of clusters and determine initial cluster centers based on intuition and experience, optimizing initial distances or selecting constant interval pieces (Milewska et al. 2013).

There was a proposal to improvise adaptive k-means with a reptile search algorithm (IAKmeans-RSA) which can be used for cyst segmentation and follicle detection. Finally, the classification is carried out using the Deep Neural Network (DNN) technique. The suggested method successfully identified PCOS using cyst detection from input photos. The algorithm's efficiency when compared to existing methods demonstrates that the suggested model is superior at segmenting and diagnosing PCOS (Sheikdavood and Ponni Bala 2023).

7.2.3 Density-Based Spatial Clustering of Applications with Noise (DBSCAN) Algorithm

DBSCAN is a well-known technique for density-based clustering since it can detect groups of various forms and handle noisy datasets (Dai and Lin 2012). The DBSCAN clustering method uses a single input parameter to identify clusters with huge spatial datasets based on local density in the database. Additionally, this method identifies outliers and noise in data. At this point, the DBSCAN clustering method provides accurate decisions for the consequences (Pasin and Ankarali 2015).

A study was conducted to detect patterns in human papillomavirus-positive women from southern Ecuador. Clustering analysis was performed on a dataset of 143 HPV patients using the DBSCAN and PAM (partition around medoids) algorithms. The results demonstrated variances based on marital status; most married and divorced women aged 30–51 have HSIL (high-grade squamous intraepithelial lesion) cytology results, while most single women aged 19–29 have LSIL (low-grade squamous intraepithelial lesion) cytology results. This shows that unmarried young women, unlike married women, prioritize cervical cancer prevention and control (Reátegui et al. 2022).

7.2.4 Gaussian-Based Mixed Model Algorithm

A Gaussian mixture model is a probabilistic framework that assumes that all data points are generated by a combination of a finite number of Gaussian distributions with unknown parameters. Mixture models can be thought of as a generalization of k-means clustering that includes information on the data's covariance structure as well as the latent Gaussian centers (Pasin and Ankarali 2015).

7.3 Preprocessing Steps Required to Prepare Reproductive Data for Clustering Analysis

The preprocessing stage of the data can involve several techniques such as scaling and normalization, transformation and projection, cleaning, and data reduction (Frigui 2004). Operational data preprocessing involves five steps: data reduction, cleaning, scaling, transformation, and partitioning. Data cleaning improves data quality by imputation of missing values and outliers. Two-dimensional data tables record building operational data, with row-wise and column-wise data reduction for minimizing dimensions and computing expenses (Fan et al. 2021).

7.3.1 Techniques for Feature Selection, Dimensionality Reduction, and Data Transformation to Enhance the Quality and Effectiveness of Clustering Results

7.3.1.1 Feature Selection for Improving Clustering Results

By identifying the subset of features that best describes the data, feature selection is used to reduce the dimensionality impact on the dataset. It filters out redundant and unnecessary features from the input data and chooses the crucial and pertinent aspects for the mining assignment (Zebari et al. 2020). Feature selection techniques include filtering, embedding, wrapping, hybridization, and ensemble methods (Zebari et al. 2020).

7.3.1.2 Dimensionality Reduction for Improving Quality and Effectiveness of Clustering

The dimensionality reduction problem of high-dimensional data is a major barrier in the modern era of healthcare and related study fields because it involves many variables that generate complicated data matrices. The need to improve data prediction, analysis, and visualization through dimension reduction of complicated data is rapidly increasing (Ray et al. 2021).

Feature extraction and selection reduce dimensions in machine learning and data mining but can affect learning quality and memory usage. Clustering is computationally costly.

7.3.1.3 Data Transformation for Enhancing the Quality of Dataset by Rescaling and Transforming

Data transformation is essential for Euclidean Distance, K-Nearest-Neighbor, k-Means, and PCA. Techniques include standardization, normalization, spectral clustering, and DipScaling and Dip Transformation. A study showed that Euclidean distance-optimized data transformation outperformed classical methods in a genomic dataset, suggesting it as a better alternative to z-standardization for multivariate data analysis (Schelling and Plant 2020).

7.4 Evaluation and Validation of Clustering Results

The performance evaluation could be computed using evaluation metrics that do not require ground truth labels to determine the clustering algorithm's efficiency. Three evaluation metrics are frequently used: Silhouette score, Calinski Harabasz index, and Davies-Bouldin index (Ogbuabor and Ugwoke 2018).

- **Silhouette score:**
- To examine the distance between the clusters created by the algorithm, silhouette analysis may be employed. One can compute the distance between the cluster using many distance metrics, including Euclidean, Manhattan, Minkowski, and Hamming. The average silhouette coefficient applied to each sample is what the silhouette score gives back (Ogbuabor and Ugwoke 2018).
- **Calinski Harabasz index:**
- The variance ratio is the foundation of the Calinski Harabasz index. The ratio between two parameters between cluster dispersion and within-cluster diffusion is computed. The quality of the clustering increases with the index (Wang and Xu 2019).
- **Davies-Bouldin index:**
- The width-cluster and between-cluster distances idea forms the basis of the Davies Bouldin index. Determining how many clusters the data points should be named in is a popular usage for it. It differs from the other two in that this index should have a low value. Consequently, lowering the DB index is the primary goal (Wang and Xu 2019).

Researchers found three papers on sexual health literacy and one Iranian questionnaire, which was the only local tool to assess Iranian people's SHELA in an adult urban population in Tehran, demonstrating strong internal correlation reliability (Panahi et al. 2022).

7.4.1 Description of Techniques for Evaluating the Compactness, Separation, and Stability of Clusters

Despite its appeal and diverse domains, diverse clustering algorithms are widely used in research due to the challenge of establishing a single effective strategy and the need for validity assessments using recognized standards (Halkidi and Vazirgiannis 2008).

Two standards that are generally accepted as adequate for gauging the effectiveness of data partitioning are:

- **Compactness:**
- The patterns inside a cluster must be distinct from patterns found in other clusters while still being comparable to one another. A cluster's compactness can be inferred from the variance of its patterns (Omran et al. 2007)
- **Separating:**
- Groups ought to be kept well apart from one another. Cluster separation is indicated by the Euclidean distance between cluster centroids (Omran et al. 2007). This study proposes the CDbw cluster validity index, which evaluates the compactness and separation of clusters created using a clustering algorithm. Rather of using a single representative point to represent each cluster, CDbw represents clusters of any shape with an efficient number of points. Complete implementation and testing results validate the validity index's reliability and demonstrate that its performance is competitive when compared to numerous others (Halkidi and Vazirgiannis 2008).

7.5 Interpreting, Understanding, and Visualizing the Methods

Cluster analysis involves exploring data patterns without strict user expectations. Essential cluster properties, like high-density regions divided from lower-density ones, are challenging to convert into statistics. Visual validation is crucial in cluster analysis, as it matches discernible patterns in data and reasonable presumptions for the chosen clustering technique (Ullmann et al. 2022).

Plots displaying raw data can evaluate trends but may rely on variables or dimension reduction. Clustering-based plots, like heatmaps or discriminant projections, highlight data patterns but may overestimate clustering validity or interpret erroneous patterns (Tellaroli et al. 2016).

7.6 Role of Men in Safeguarding Reproductive Health

The improved communication within couples and advantages for reproductive health can result from joint counselling between women receiving antenatal care (ANC) coverage services and their partners. The couples in South Africa and India may choose from same-sex group counselling, individual counselling, or joint counselling during prenatal care visits (Mukherjee et al. 2019). Several participants held the views that having sex before the age of 18 was dangerous, that having sex more than three times a week was dangerous, and that losing sperm could cause physical harm or sexual dysfunction. The survey conducted by Mukherjee et al. (2019) found that 47.1% of men and 34.5% of women believed that using a condom reduces pleasure. Similarly, 58.0% of men and 65.8% of women expressed their agreement that sex education should be mandated. In addition, 74.6% of men and

71.6% of women expressed agreement with the notion that males should abstain from sexual activity until marriage, while 82.9% of men and 80.4% of women expressed agreement with the notion that women should abstain from sexual activity until marriage. The survey findings also indicate that 60.7% of men and 47.6% of women expressed agreement with the notion that engaging in sexual activity more than three times a week is detrimental. Moreover, a majority of men (67.1%) and women (58.9%) agreed that engaging in sexual behavior during menstruation is detrimental to males (Mukherjee et al. 2019).

Men's desire for understanding spouses' needs is evident in combined counselling, but challenges persist. New Delhi's joint counselling increased attendance, improved communication, and postpartum contraception, leading to its expansion to all insurance facilities (Frontiers in Reproductive 2009).

7.7 Role of Government and Nongovernment Organizations in Reproductive Health

The cluster strategy aims to enhance sexual and reproductive health effectiveness by identifying interconnected concerns and forming 11 clusters. Chaired by UN agencies, NGOs, or national governments, these clusters focus on various sectors, including telecommunications, education, shelter, agriculture, and early recovery. Clustering analysis can identify similar subpopulations and develop targeted interventions (IASC 2006).

7.8 Cluster Analysis in Reproductive Health Studies

The health disparities between social groups can be caused by disparities in access to healthcare. These disparities are not always considered in interventions aimed at improving health outcomes and granting everyone access to healthcare. Worldwide, women are subject to unequal access to healthcare services (Ogundele et al. 2020). The survival and growth of the female population are impacted by women's health, as is the well-being of family members, particularly the following generation. According to a US cohort research, moms who led healthy lifestyles before becoming pregnant—including maintaining a normal weight, eating well, exercising regularly, not smoking, and drinking alcohol in moderation—had better offspring. Nonetheless, reproductive health and fertility intentions have been the main subjects of most of the research on women of childbearing age (He et al. 2023). This chapter explores clustered analysis's use in reproductive health studies, discussing different algorithms and selecting the right one for a study, and providing examples of its application in various reproductive health themes.

7.9 Prophylaxis

Contraception is the use of artificial or natural methods to prevent pregnancy, and should be easily accessible, affordable, and provided by qualified healthcare professionals. It reduces maternal and infant mortality, improves newborn and child health, and enhances girls' educational opportunities (WHO 2017).

The clustering analysis has been used to recognize subpopulations of women with diverse contraceptive use patterns and inclinations. This data can be studied further to develop targeted interventions to extend contraceptive use and decrease unintended pregnancy (WHO 2017).

Additionally, improved condom use among all users of highly and moderately effective contraceptive methods is necessary, according to a study comparing the use of condoms with various techniques including LARC (to long-acting reversible contraceptives) users. Improving dual protection among adolescents is crucial for achieving pregnancy and STI (sexually transmitter infections) prevention goals (Justin Landegger et al. 2011). During the acute and more stable phases of a humanitarian crisis, the key sexual and reproductive health activities include obstetric emergency care, initiatives to promote safe motherhood, reduction in the spread of HIV, STI and HIV prevention and treatment, family preparation, improvements in GBV protection, strengthening of GBV reporting procedures, emergency contraception for GBV survivors as well as psychological and social support, and more (WHO 1999).

A study using US National Health and Nutrition Examination Surveys reveals a cluster of common chronic illnesses affecting women with infected urinary tracts. Cardiovascular disease is common in all age groups, while pulmonary disease, particularly asthma, affects all women in one cluster. Clinical recommendations for UI should consider treatment-related adverse effects (Markland et al. 2018).

Scientists studied data from 967 AGYW in South Africa who started oral PrEP. They found a high rate of early discontinuation, with only a small percentage using it for more than 4 months. However, a significant number returned and restarted PrEP, with factors like age, contraceptive use, and initiation location influencing restarts (Martin et al. 2023).

7.10 Fertility

As communities transition from naturally occurring to artificially created offspring, intentional marital fertility control increases. Despite increased use of contraceptives, induced abortion remains common. This affects marriage and postpartum infertility. A total of 30–75% of male infertile individuals have no primary cause, leading to idiopathic or unexplained infertility (Schubert et al. 2022).

A more profound view can be given through new analysis methods like cluster analysis and machine learning. These creative studies can reveal previously undetected patterns in data that andrologists may find challenging to identify but which these techniques make obvious (Schubert et al. 2022).

There is no evidence of global fertility convergence after WWII, and countries can be classified into different clubs based on their fertility rates. Additionally, the study suggests that factors such as economic development, population diversity, genetic distance, and transition to agriculture can affect the barriers to fertility decline (Papagni 2023).

The improved understanding of fertility issues and cutting-edge medical technology, such as assisted reproductive technologies like in vitro fertilization (IVF), are among the interventions for fertility care. Providing fertility care also presents a significant chance to interact with guys, who are typically less inclined to seek medical attention or have sexual health-related conversations (WHO 2017).

A 2021 study in Burundi identified six distinct clusters based on contraceptive and pregnancy behaviors, using Burundi DHS 2016–2017 contraceptive calendar data. The approach helps develop adaptable strategies to meet women's diverse fertility needs, identifying traits related to family planning, fertility, and demographics that are connected to these clusters (MacQuarrie et al. 2021).

7.11 Pregnancy

Cluster analysis helps identify pregnant females at higher risk for preeclamptic syndromes, preterm labor, or premature labor, enabling targeted interventions to mitigate these risks.

A survey of 535 disabled women in central Gondar zone revealed that only one in three of them used SRH services. To improve utilization, optimal family size, sexual activity at the recommended age, travel autonomy, candid communication, partner living, and media exposure are recommended. All parties involved must work together to increase SRH service usage (Rade et al. 2023).

A study of 293 young women found cluster analysis of anxiety, sadness, stress, and quality of life, revealing high-risk groups with lower anxiety and depression levels, suggesting appropriate care can improve mental health (Lim et al. 2015).

A cross-sectional study of 557 pregnant women revealed a range of psychosomatic problems, with varying symptom presentations at different phases. The investigation sheds light on the symptom clusters experienced by pregnant women (Zhang et al. 2023).

Although most of the kids belonged to the "processed" cluster, there were some differences in the kids' dietary clusters based on their mothers' dietary clusters (Table 7.1). A third of the offspring of mothers in the "fruit and vegetables" cluster during pregnancy belonged to the "plant-based" cluster; by comparison, less than a fifth of the offspring of mothers in the other two groups were in the "plant-based" cluster (Freitas-Vilela et al. 2017).

Table 7.1 Depiction of an example of comparison of cluster membership of pregnant women to cluster membership of their 7-year-old descendants

Pattern of expectant mother's diet				
Childs food regimen	White bread/coffee[a] (%)	Meat and potato[a] (%)	Fruits and vegetables[a] (%)	Total (%)
Based on plants[a]	17.3	19.4	35.3	25.1
Conventional British[a]	24.6	26.7	23.1	24.4
Finished/processed[a]	58.1	53.9	41.6	50.5
Total	100.0	100.0	100.0	100.0

[a]Dietary patterns are clustered between mothers and children according to a chi-square test <0.001

7.12 Maternal and Child Health

The study used clustering analysis to identify subpopulations of women and children at high risk for poor health outcomes, examining factors like perinatal and demography, Bayley scores, and CBCL scores, and determining separate child groups.

A cluster randomized trial in Bulgan, Mongolia, evaluated the effectiveness of a translated MCH handbook in encouraging antenatal care attendance. The intervention group received the handbook during their first prenatal visit, while the control group received it 9 months later (Mori et al. 2015).

A quasi-experimental study was conducted between 2015 and 2020 using the Find Link Treat and Retain (FLTR) approach, community-owned initiatives, and four control clusters to examine the effects of EHC implementation on maternal and child health indices. Results showed comprehensive improvement in service use and accessibility (Esamai et al. 2023).

Women in cluster groups 1 and 3 were less likely than those in cluster groups 1 and 2 to have had care from a doctor, nurse/midwife, and auxiliary staff (Fig. 7.1). Additionally, they had a higher probability of having been exposed to mother-to-child transmission (MTCT) of AIDS talks, being offered an AIDS test at ANC, testing positive for the virus, giving birth in a government or public facility, caesarean delivery, receiving timely health check-ups after delivery, and receiving delivery checks before being released from the facility (Ayanore et al. 2016).

A study found that parental support is crucial for treating excessive infant crying, but many parents feel unsupported by healthcare professionals. The study found that mothers of infants with medical conditions rated healthcare more effective but were more dissatisfied. Effective reassurance and sensitivity to family needs are essential (Van der Veek and van Rosmalen 2023).

Aceh Province, Indonesia, has a positive correlation with maternal and child health services, including blood-supplementing tablets, first visit coverage, and obstetric management. The study identifies three districts based on quality of services and suggests enhancing these services through community involvement, observation, and assessment (Whidden et al. 2023).

Table 7.2 demonstrates few metabolites have the potential to function as biomarkers for the early identification of noncommunicable diseases in women and

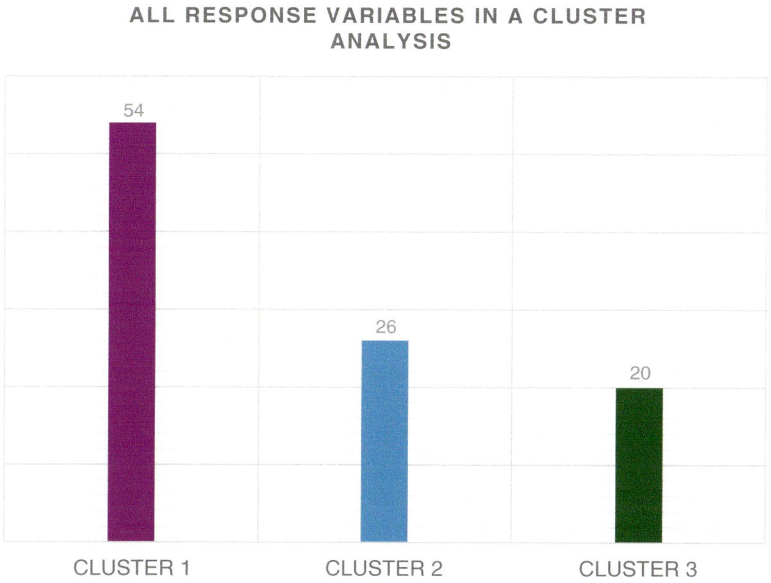

Fig. 7.1 Illustrates the cluster analysis and the general distribution of the Ghanaian respondents that were analyzed. Cluster 2 denotes less adequate care, Cluster 3 indicates least adequate worse treatment, while Cluster 1 represents appropriate care (Ayanore et al. 2016)

Table 7.2 Potential biomarkers for metabolites linked to illnesses that are not transmissible that impact children and their mothers (Cerf 2023)

Illness, disease or disorder	Supplement	Inadequacy
Poly cystic ovarian syndrome	Trimethylamine N-oxide (TMAO) valine, isoleucine, leucine etc.	–
Mental disorder	Isoleucine	Valine, leucine
Cancer	Myristic acid, palmitic acid, PDAC Adrenic acid, arachidonic acid, linoleic acid	Creatine, succinate, taurine, tryptophane glutamate, isoleucine, proline
Obesity	Increased in kids with a lot of visceral fat Lysophosopholipids (LysoPC 14:0, LysoPC 16:3, LysoPC 16:1, LysoPC 16:0, LysoPS 21:1, LysoPS 25:6 and LysoPA 23:1), dimethylarginine, diacylglycerol. PC (18:1/16:0), PC plasmalogen (34:1)	Elevated in young people with less visceral fat Lysophosphatidylserine (LysoPSs), lysophosphosphatidic acid (LysoPA), sphingomyelin
Diabetes during pregnancy	Arginine	3-Hydroxy-isovalerylcarnitine, glycine
Diabetes	Glutamic acid; glutamine,7-methylguanine, aspartate, cystine, glutamate, etc.	Alanine, serine
Preeclampsia	Glutamate; palmitoleic acid, 3-phosphoglycerate, arachidonic acid, etc.	Lipoxin A4
Heart-related condition	Choline, trimethylamine, betaine, etc.	Proline, succinate, taurine, creatine, glutamate, isoleucine, tryptophane

children, which can improve prognosis by predicting pre-disease states, risk factors, and beginning of these conditions.

7.13 Conclusion

The current chapter looks at the use of clustered analysis in reproductive health studies, the different types of clustered algorithms that can be used, and the factors to consider when choosing a clustered algorithm for a specific study. This chapter indicates that women who are of reproductive age generally have good overall health. Nonetheless, a sizable segment of women continues to fall short in certain areas, including self-rated health, disease, and mental health. It was found that lifestyle was the most significant influencing factor on the overall health status of women who are reproductive age. This could potentially provide areas for future research and development of interventions aimed at improving the health of women globally. In summary, the use of the health systems approach in healthcare delivery results in a significant enhancement in health indices and the utilization and accessibility of health services.

References

Ayanore MA, Pavlova M, Groot W (2016) Focused maternity care in Ghana: results of a cluster analysis. BMC Health Serv Res 16:395. https://doi.org/10.1186/s12913-016-1654-5

Cerf ME (2023) Maternal and child health, non-communicable diseases and metabolites. Metabolites 13:756. https://doi.org/10.3390/metabo13060756

Dai B-R, Lin I-C (2012) Efficient map/reduce-based DBSCAN algorithm with optimized data partition. In: 2012 IEEE fifth international conference on cloud computing. IEEE, Honolulu, pp 59–66

Dapas M, Lin FTJ, Nadkarni GN et al (2020) Distinct subtypes of polycystic ovary syndrome with novel genetic associations: an unsupervised, phenotypic clustering analysis. PLoS Med 17:e1003132. https://doi.org/10.1371/journal.pmed.1003132

Esamai F, Mwangi A, Nangami M et al (2023) Maternal and child health indicators in primary healthcare facilities: findings in a health systems quasi-experimental study in western Kenya. Dialogues in Health 2:100133. https://doi.org/10.1016/j.dialog.2023.100133

Fan C, Chen M, Wang X et al (2021) A review on data preprocessing techniques toward efficient and reliable knowledge discovery from building operational data. Front Energy Res 9. https://doi.org/10.3389/fenrg.2021.652801

Freitas-Vilela AA, Smith ADAC, Kac G et al (2017) Dietary patterns by cluster analysis in pregnant women: relationship with nutrient intakes and dietary patterns in 7-year-old offspring. Matern Child Nutr 13:e12353. https://doi.org/10.1111/mcn.12353

Frigui H (2004) Pre-processing for data clustering. In: IEEE annual meeting of the fuzzy information, 2004. Processing NAFIPS '04, vol 2. IEEE, Banff, pp 967–972

Frontiers in Reproductive Health (2009) Gender and reproductive health services: putting gender perspective into practice. Population Council

Halkidi M, Vazirgiannis M (2008) A density-based cluster validity approach using multi-representatives. Pattern Recogn Lett 29:773–786. https://doi.org/10.1016/j.patrec.2007.12.011

He L, Li S-T, Qin M-X et al (2023) Unsupervised clustering analysis of comprehensive health status and its influencing factors on women of childbearing age: a cross-sectional study

from a province in central China. BMC Public Health 23:2206. https://doi.org/10.1186/s12889-023-17096-3
Inter-Agency Standing Committee (2006) IASC guidance note on using the cluster approach to strengthen humanitarian response. In: Refworld. https://www.refworld.org/policy/legalguidance/iasc/2006/en/40930. Accessed 27 Mar 2024
Landegger J, Hau M, Kaducu F et al (2011) Strengths and weaknesses of the humanitarian Cluster Approach in relation to sexual and reproductive health services in northern Uganda. Int Health 3:108–114. https://doi.org/10.1016/j.inhe.2011.03.005
Lim MSC, Zhang X-D, Kennedy E et al (2015) Sexual and reproductive health knowledge, contraception uptake, and factors associated with unmet need for modern contraception among adolescent female sex workers in China. PLoS One 10:e0115435. https://doi.org/10.1371/journal.pone.0115435
MacQuarrie KLD, Allen C, Gemmill A (2021) Demographic and fertility characteristics of contraceptive clusters in Burundi. Stud Fam Plan 52:415–438. https://doi.org/10.1111/sifp.12179
Markland AD, Vaughan CP, Okosun IS et al (2018) Cluster analysis of multiple chronic conditions associated with urinary incontinence among women in the USA. BJU Int 122:1041–1048. https://doi.org/10.1111/bju.14246
Martin CE, Cox LA, Nongena P et al (2023) Patterns of HIV pre-exposure prophylaxis use among adolescent girls and young women accessing routine sexual and reproductive health services in South Africa. J Adolesc Health 73:S81–S91. https://doi.org/10.1016/j.jadohealth.2023.08.004
Milewska AJ, Jankowska D, Cwalina U et al (2013) Analyzing outcomes of intrauterine insemination treatment by application of cluster analysis or Kohonen neural networks. Stud Log Gramm Rhetor 35:7–25. https://doi.org/10.2478/slgr-2013-0041
Mori R, Yonemoto N, Noma H et al (2015) The Maternal and Child Health (MCH) handbook in Mongolia: a cluster-randomized, controlled trial. PLoS One 10:e0119772. https://doi.org/10.1371/journal.pone.0119772
Mukherjee A, Gopalakrishnan R, Thangadurai P et al (2019) Knowledge and attitudes toward sexual health and common sexual practices among college students—a survey from Vellore, Tamil Nadu, India. Indian J Psychol Med 41:348–356. https://doi.org/10.4103/IJPSYM.IJPSYM_441_18
Ogbuabor G, Ugwoke FN (2018) Clustering algorithm for a healthcare dataset using Silhouette score value. IJCSIT 10:27–37. https://doi.org/10.5121/ijcsit.2018.10203
Ogundele OJ, Pavlova M, Groot W (2020) Patterns of access to reproductive health services in Ghana and Nigeria: results of a cluster analysis. BMC Public Health 20:549. https://doi.org/10.1186/s12889-020-08724-3
Omran MGH, Engelbrecht AP, Salman A (2007) An overview of clustering methods. IDA 11:583–605. https://doi.org/10.3233/IDA-2007-11602
Panahi R, Dehghankar L, Amjadian M (2022) Investigating the structural validity and reliability of the sexual health literacy for adults (SHELA) questionnaire among a sample of women in Qazvin, Iran. BMC Womens Health 22:524. https://doi.org/10.1186/s12905-022-02112-2
Papagni E (2023) Long-term barriers to global fertility convergence. J Popul Econ 36:431–470. https://doi.org/10.1007/s00148-022-00895-0
Pasin Ö, Ankarali H (2015) Usage of Kernel K-Means and DBSCAN cluster algorıthms in health studies: an application. Clin Res Trial 1:63–69. https://doi.org/10.15761/CRT.1000116
Rada C (2014) Sexual behaviour and sexual and reproductive health education: a cross-sectional study in Romania. Reprod Health 11:48. https://doi.org/10.1186/1742-4755-11-48
Rade BK, Tamiru AT, Aynalem GL et al (2023) Prevalence and factors associated with sexual and reproductive health services use among reproductive age women with disabilities: a community based cross-sectional study. BMC Womens Health 23:215. https://doi.org/10.1186/s12905-023-02373-5
Ray P, Reddy SS, Banerjee T (2021) Various dimension reduction techniques for high dimensional data analysis: a review. Artif Intell Rev 54:3473–3515. https://doi.org/10.1007/s10462-020-09928-0

Reátegui R, Bautista-Valarezo E, Ortega-Vivanco M et al (2022) Comparison of clusters algorithms to identify patterns in information related to cervical cancer. In: Rocha A, Adeli H, Dzemyda G, Moreira F (eds) Information systems and technologies. Springer International Publishing, Cham, pp 403–412

Schelling B, Plant C (2020) Dataset-transformation: improving clustering by enhancing the structure with DipScaling and DipTransformation. Knowl Inf Syst 62:457–484. https://doi.org/10.1007/s10115-019-01388-5

Schubert M, Krenz H, Sansone A et al (2022) O-248 Cluster analysis of men with idiopathic and unexplained male infertility identifies FSHB Genotype as relevant diagnostic parameter. Hum Reprod 37(deac106):030. https://doi.org/10.1093/humrep/deac106.030

Sheikdavood K, Ponni Bala M (2023) Polycystic ovary cyst segmentation using adaptive K-means with reptile search algorith. ITC 52:85–99. https://doi.org/10.5755/j01.itc.52.1.32096

Tellaroli P, Bazzi M, Donato M et al (2016) Cross-clustering: a partial clustering algorithm with automatic estimation of the number of clusters. PLoS One 11:e0152333. https://doi.org/10.1371/journal.pone.0152333

Ullmann T, Hennig C, Boulesteix A (2022) Validation of cluster analysis results on validation data: a systematic framework. WIREs Data Min Knowl 12:e1444. https://doi.org/10.1002/widm.1444

Van Der Veek SMC, Van Rosmalen L (2023) Maternal satisfaction with professional health care for excessive infant crying: does it meet maternal needs? Early Child Dev Care 193:602–615. https://doi.org/10.1080/03004430.2022.2130903

Wang X, Xu Y (2019) An improved index for clustering validation based on Silhouette index and Calinski-Harabasz index. IOP Conf Ser: Mater Sci Eng 569:052024. https://doi.org/10.1088/1757-899X/569/5/052024

Whidden C, Kayentao K, Koné N et al (2023) Effects of proactive vs fixed community health care delivery on child health and access to care: a cluster randomised trial secondary endpoint analysis. J Glob Health 13:04047. https://doi.org/10.7189/jogh.13.04047

WHO (2017) Sexual health and its linkages to reproductive health: an operational approach. https://www.who.int/publications-detail-redirect/9789241151288. Accessed 27 Mar 2024

World Health Organization (1999) Reproductive Health in refugee situations: an inter agency field manual (UNHCR/WHO/UNFPA). In: UNHCR India. https://www.unhcr.org/in/media/reproductive-health-refugee-situations-inter-agency-field-manual-unhcr-who-unfpa. Accessed 27 Mar 2024

Zebari R, Abdulazeez A, Zeebaree D et al (2020) A comprehensive review of dimensionality reduction techniques for feature selection and feature extraction. JASTT 1:56–70. https://doi.org/10.38094/jastt1224

Zhang B, Zhang L, Chen Q et al (2023) Harnessing artificial intelligence to improve clinical trial design. Commun Med 3:191. https://doi.org/10.1038/s43856-023-00425-3

Leveraging Natural Language Processing for Enhanced Pharmacovigilance in Reproductive Health

8

Manjunath Ramanna Lamani, K. Padmaja, V. Asha, M. Somesha, B. L. Shilpa, and M. Anand

Abstract

Natural Language Processing (NLP) stands at the forefront of contemporary pharmacovigilance and pharmaceutical datasets, offering a robust framework for monitoring drug safety and identifying adverse events with unprecedented efficiency. In the complex terrain of reproductive health, this technical paper investigates how NLP extends beyond conventional methodologies, addressing the unique surveillance demands of contraception, fertility treatments, and maternal health. We detail the versatile applications of NLP in recognizing and categorizing side effects from reproductive health drugs, drawing on diverse data streams such as patient narratives, electronic health records, and online social interactions. This approach makes the drug safety monitoring process faster and more effective, greatly improving the ability to spot safety concerns. Delving further, the paper presents an in-depth analysis of signal detection techniques within reproductive health, leveraging advanced NLP algorithms to sift through extensive data troves. These algorithms are adept at discerning intricate patterns and trends, highlighting medication safety issues, and informing a nuanced risk-

M. R. Lamani (✉)
Department of Computer Science and Engineering, CHRIST (Deemed to be University), Bengaluru, India
e-mail: manjunath.lamani@res.christuniversity.in

K. Padmaja · M. Anand
ISE Department, Engineering Campus, GSSS Institute of Engineering & Technology for Women, Mysore, India

V. Asha · M. Somesha
Department of Computer Science and Engineering, Government SKSJ Technological Institute, Bangalore, India

B. L. Shilpa
Department of CSE, ATME College of Engineering, Mysore, India

A. Sengupta et al. (eds.), *Data-Driven Reproductive Health*,
https://doi.org/10.1007/978-981-97-7451-7_8

benefit calculus that enhances drug safety protocols. The untapped potential of NLP is also highlighted as a transformative force within the dynamic field of pharmacovigilance, aiding healthcare practitioners and regulatory authorities in pinpointing safety risks and fostering evidence-based decision-making. NLP's capacity to distill vast data into actionable intelligence is a pivotal advancement, enabling more responsive regulatory measures and promoting patient safety. Additionally, this paper delineates how NLP can be instrumental in shaping regulatory frameworks, quickening risk management processes, and expediting the update of medical guidelines and drug labels. Our research provides tangible illustrations through case studies that underscore NLP's efficacy in fortifying reproductive health pharmacovigilance and pharmaceutical datasets and enhancing patient safety and public health in sensitive domains such as contraception and maternity care. Ultimately, the paper positions NLP as a revolutionary paradigm in the field, catalyzing the early detection of safety signals, streamlining risk assessment, and informing regulatory actions with a comprehensive linguistic and textual analysis foundation. This work showcases NLP's pivotal role in transforming the pharmacovigilance and pharmaceutical dataset. It underlines its significance in ensuring that medications are safer and more effectively tailored to meet the needs of patients and the broader healthcare ecosystem.

Keywords

NLP · Pharmacovigilance · Drug safety monitoring · Adverse event detection Patient safety enhancement · Evidence-based regulatory actions

8.1 Introduction

Employing Natural Language Processing (NLP) in both reproductive health and pharmacovigilance significantly enhances healthcare outcomes. In reproductive health, NLP accelerates the analysis of health records and digital platforms, unveiling critical health trends and enabling the development of personalized, accessible educational materials. Such tools, including chatbots, offer instant, reliable counsel and support decision-making with advanced analytics, ensuring a private and inclusive approach to healthcare. Similarly, in the pharmacovigilance sector, NLP excels in detecting Adverse Drug Reactions (ADRs) early by efficiently parsing through extensive data sources. It streamlines adverse event reporting, aiding healthcare providers and patients in contributing to safer drug use. This dual application of NLP not only fortifies patient safety but also bolsters the quality of healthcare data, driving forward the improvement of healthcare services and drug safety management.

Pharmacovigilance is essential in monitoring and preventing Adverse Drug Reactions (ADRs), which are critical for balancing the benefits and risks of medications post-market release. This process is key to ensuring drug safety and efficacy, given the limitations of pre-release data on new medications. ADRs pose serious health risks and can incur substantial economic costs, emphasizing the need for effective pharmacovigilance to manage the trade-off between drug accessibility and safety (WHO 2017). Additionally, the significant investment in drug development necessitates efficient market entry of safe drugs and continuous post-market safety monitoring. Despite its importance, the traditional pharmacovigilance system faces challenges in cost and timeliness, potentially missing unreported ADRs. Advanced pharmacovigilance tools aim to improve ADR monitoring and safety evaluations, making the process more responsive and cost-effective (Pharmacovigilance 2020; Schmider et al. 2019).

Social media's emergence has revolutionized communication, especially in health information exchange, with more patients seeking health guidance online due to limited doctor availability, a preference for involvement in health decisions, and the anonymity of digital spaces (Umefjord et al. 2003; Dickerson et al. 2006; Tyson 2000; Gerber and Eiser 2001). Adverse Drug Reactions (ADRs) pose a significant public health challenge, with millions of severe cases reported annually. While drug approvals are based on clinical trial outcomes showing benefits over risks, post-marketing surveillance, such as the FDA's MedWatch program, is crucial for monitoring ongoing safety. These programs depend on voluntary reports from health professionals and patients to catch adverse events early. However, the optional nature of these reports can delay the recognition of critical safety concerns, highlighting the importance of prompt ADR detection systems (Lazarou et al. 1998; ADRs 2009; Almenoff et al. 2007; Hochberg et al. 2007; Hauben and Bate 2009; Harpaz et al. 2010).

8.2 Related Work

Health forums on social media are becoming increasingly popular for patients to discuss illnesses and share health concerns. Traditional statistical topic analysis faces challenges due to the expanding volume of Internet data. This study introduces a novel approach using document clustering to automatically identify topics in online health forums, focusing on lung cancer, breast cancer, and diabetes discussions. Prevalent topics include symptoms, testing, prescriptions, treatments, and general health concerns. The study also addresses the difficulty of early Adverse Drug Reaction (ADR) detection during medical treatment, using a text mining approach with Hidden Markov Model (HMM) classification that outperforms the baseline. The findings underscore the potential of online healthcare forums for early ADR identification, contributing to improved drug safety (Sampathkumar et al. 2014). In the EU, the Pharmacovigilance Risk Assessment Committee (PRAC) oversees pharmaceutical risk management, emphasizing patient-centric strategies to minimize adverse drug reactions and enhance drug accessibility. Proactive pharmacovigilance integrates throughout the pharmaceutical life cycle, involving high-innovation firms in pre-release implementation. Source analysis with NLP automation is crucial, and our study addresses the lack of Russian-language medical datasets, presenting a method for extracting entity relations from Russian medical texts. Comparisons demonstrate the method's effectiveness, surpassing existing models in accuracy (Santoro et al. 2017). Artificial Intelligence (AI) is advancing rapidly across sectors, including social networks, with applications in pattern recognition models. Our study introduces the Hopfield Feedback Neural Network (HFNN) pattern recognition system, achieving high accuracy in the presence of noise. In language learning, we propose a novel approach using interlanguage word similarity and part-of-speech (POS) tagging to train and evaluate Neural Machine Translation (NMT) systems. Our method, assessed across multiple languages, outperforms existing models in terms of BLEU, Score, Precision, and METEOR (Sboev et al. 2022; De Oliveira and Tadeu Braga 2020; Ganesh et al. 2021; Xu et al. 2021; Peters et al. 2018).

This study explores advancements in various language models and their applications in diverse domains. BIBERT, a bilingual pre-trained language model, demonstrates superior translation results with contextualized embeddings. Another research emphasizes the effectiveness of feed-forward neural network learning models over N-gram models for author categorization. A deep Bidirectional Language Model (biLM) enhances natural language processing tasks, achieving significant improvements. In neural machine translation, a local attention mechanism outperforms dropout-based systems, and an ensemble model excels in English-to-German translation. BioBERT, trained on biomedical data, outperforms BERT in biomedical text mining tasks. In Russian text mining, a corpus with connected items is introduced, and XLM-RoBERTa aids in extracting entity relations with high accuracy. BioALBERT, derived from transformers, outperforms existing models in medical tasks. Beyond language models, innovative research utilizes Twitter for drug-related trend detection and real-time allergy monitoring. Additionally, data mining on social media unveils insights into suicide risk factors among South Korean teens, and sentiment analysis on a marijuana-related Facebook page informs public health policymaking.

The primary approach to monitoring nationwide Drug Overdose (OD) mortality relies on Death Certificates (DCs), providing crucial details on demographics and substances involved. Unfortunately, delays in analysis arise due to forensic processes, hindering the timely tracking of drug OD trends. Recognizing Twitter's significance in discussions on health topics, this study proposes a Twitter Adverse Drug Reaction (ADR) monitoring system using supervised learning, Conditional Random Fields (CRFs), and Support Vector Machines (SVMs). Social media data mining, including sentiment analysis, proves vital in understanding emotions expressed in these discussions. The study underlines the importance of real-time monitoring of medical disorders through text analysis and machine learning on social media platforms, addressing concerns over skewed datasets and manual annotation. The broader goal is to enhance post-market drug safety monitoring, emphasizing data analytics as "the new oil" across industries (Tekin et al. 2019; Zucco et al. 2017; Akay et al. 2016; Dai et al. 2016; Dai and Wang 2019; Gräßer et al. 2018; Katragadda et al. 2015; Lin et al. 2015; Mishra et al. 2015).

In our data-driven era, effective decision-making requires integrating technology and knowledge, with statistical analysis transforming vast datasets into meaningful information. AI, machine learning, and big data have revolutionized customer-focused online marketing for businesses striving for competitive sustainability. The demand for demographic, interest, and purchase data is crucial for reaching target groups, evaluating customer behavior, and enabling effective communication. Strategic decisions increasingly rely on data, and automation through machine learning contributes to accurate decision-making (Tekin et al. 2019). While recognizing the potential benefits of AI, Big Data, and Automation in surgery, caution is advised, emphasizing the need for smarter training for surgeons to oversee autonomous surgeries without compromising manual skills (Wall and Krummel 2020). This essay explores big data comprehensively, critiquing its hasty corporate adoption without sufficient philosophical discussion and advocating for scholarly monitoring of "big data" discussions. It covers various data types, including text, audio, video, and social media, with a specific focus on video analytics, and discusses anticipated developments in big data analytics, providing a thorough examination of its pros and cons (Gandomi and Haider 2015).

8.3 Materials and Methodology

8.3.1 Preprocessing

In the preprocessing of the "medicine_dataset.csv," several steps were undertaken to ensure data quality and readiness for analysis. Firstly, the "use0" column was addressed to handle missing values by replacing them with the placeholder "Unknown". Subsequently, text-cleaning techniques were applied to the same column, removing special characters, numbers, and extraneous whitespaces to enhance uniformity and coherence in the textual data. This process aimed to standardize the representation of medical uses or indications for the medications across the dataset. These preprocessing steps are essential for mitigating the impact of missing values and promoting consistency in the textual data, laying a solid foundation for subsequent analyses or machine learning tasks on the pharmacovigilance and pharmaceutical dataset.

Figure 8.1 provides a succinct summary of data incompleteness by displaying the count of missing values for each column. Concurrently, the heatmap presents a more detailed representation, highlighting the locations of missing values through yellow lines across the dataset. This combined visualization approach facilitates a comprehensive assessment of data gaps, aiding in the identification of specific columns and patterns where values are absent. The exploration of missing values plays a pivotal role in data preprocessing, enabling well-informed decisions regarding imputation strategies or column removal. Ultimately, this enhances the reliability of subsequent analyses and machine learning tasks conducted on the pharmaceutical dataset.

8.3.2 Architecture

The one-hot encoding and Natural Language Processing (NLP) techniques were applied to the pharmacovigilance and pharmaceutical dataset to transform

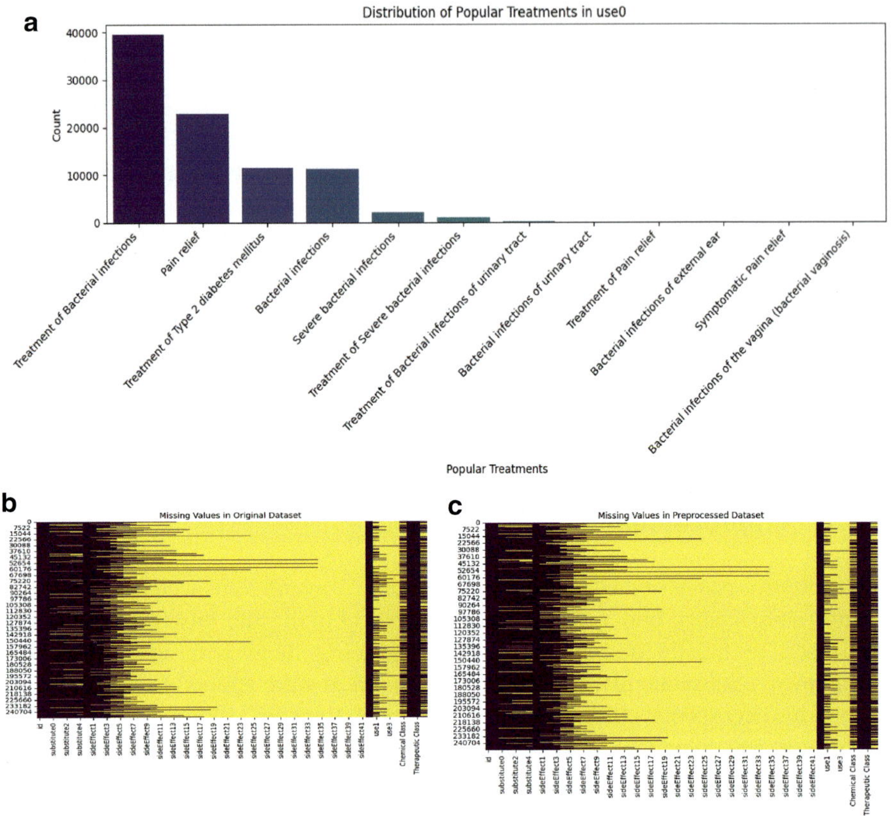

Fig. 8.1 (**a**) Bar chart of distribution of popular treatments; (**b**) Heat map missing values in the original dataset; and (**c**) Heat map missing values in the preprocessed dataset

categorical text data into a numerical format suitable for machine learning algorithms. Specifically, the columns related to chemical classes, therapeutic classes, and action classes were selected for one-hot encoding. This process involved creating binary columns for each unique category, marking the presence or absence of a specific class. Additionally, the "use0" column, which contained textual information about medical uses, underwent NLP preprocessing. Tokenization and vectorization were employed to convert the text into numerical features, allowing the incorporation of textual information in machine learning models. These encoding strategies facilitate the utilization of categorical and textual information for predictive modeling, enhancing the dataset's compatibility with various machine learning algorithms.

Feature extraction and selection processes were employed to enhance the relevance and efficiency of the pharmacovigilance and pharmaceutical dataset for subsequent analyses in Fig. 8.2. Feature extraction involved the creation of binary columns indicating the presence of specific side effects and popular treatments, offering a more granular representation of the data. Additionally, the dataset's

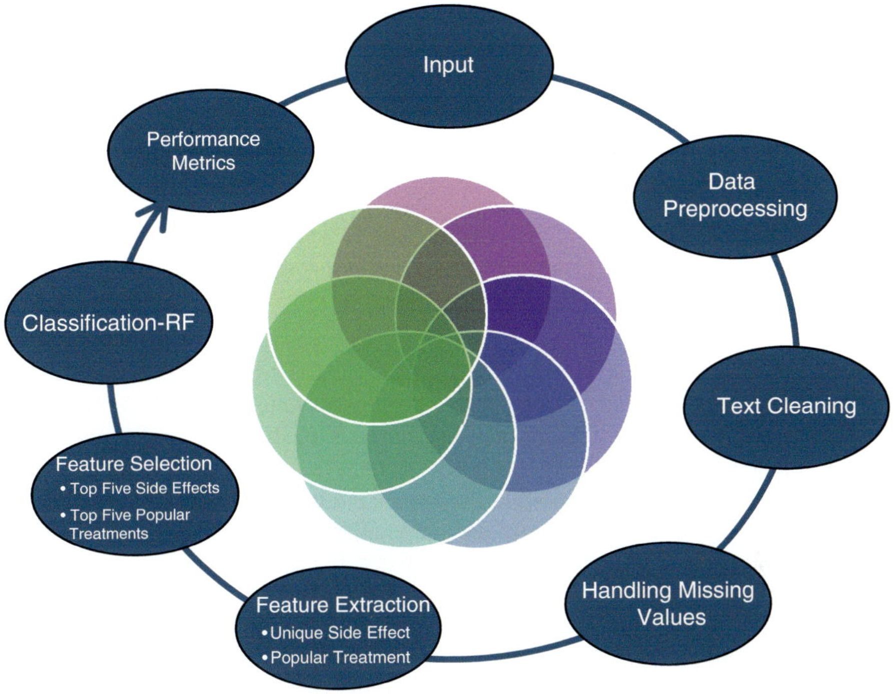

Fig. 8.2 Block diagram of the architecture (NLP data processing and classification)

features were enriched by incorporating information on the top five prevalent side effects and treatments, enhancing the representation of key factors. Feature selection, on the other hand, involves choosing a subset of features deemed most influential for modeling. In this context, the top five popular side effects and treatments were identified and retained, streamlining the dataset to focus on critical variables. These extraction and selection strategies collectively aimed to capture essential information, reduce dimensionality, and improve the dataset's utility for predictive modeling and analysis within the pharmaceutical domain.

8.4 Results and Discussion with Case Study

8.4.1 Dataset

The pharmacovigilance (A pharmacovigilance dataset focusing on reproductive health critically encompasses drug and demographic information, details of adverse drug reactions, pregnancy outcomes, clinical effectiveness, and reporting sources to assess medication safety comprehensively.) and pharmaceutical dataset (The dataset highlights key aspects of reproductive health drugs, focusing on safety, effectiveness, and usage patterns (Singh et al. 2023) consist of 248,218 entries with 58

Table 8.1 Main columns of the pharmacovigilance and pharmaceutical dataset

ID	Information
id	A unique identifier for each medication
name	The name of the medication
substitute0 to substitute4	Potential substitutes for the medication
sideEffect0 to sideEffect41	Potential side effects associated with the medication
use0 to use4	Possible medical uses or indications for the medication
Chemical Class	The chemical class to which the medication belongs
Therapeutic Class	The therapeutic class or category of the medication
Action Class	The action class of the medication

columns in Table 8.1. Each row represents information about a specific medication (https://www.kaggle.com/datasets). Here is a breakdown of the dataset columns.

The dataset includes a unique identifier for each medication, which allows for easy referencing and avoidance of confusion between drugs with similar names. Each medication has up to five listed substitutes, indicating possible alternatives for patients who may need different options due to allergies, side effects, cost, or availability. With up to 42 potential side effects listed for each medication, the dataset provides comprehensive information on the adverse reactions associated with each drug. This can be valuable for healthcare providers and patients in managing and anticipating drug safety concerns. The dataset outlines up to five medical uses for each medication, which could be used to assess the versatility of a drug or to identify drugs that could be repurposed for other indications. Grouping medications by their chemical class can reveal patterns in side effects or efficacy among drugs with similar chemical structures. The therapeutic class provides insight into the scope of diseases and conditions that the medications are designed to treat. The indication of whether a medication is habit-forming is crucial for understanding the potential for abuse and dependence. This information could be used to guide prescribing practices and patient counseling. Understanding the action class of a medication helps in knowing the mechanism by which the drug works. This can be important in predicting drug-drug interactions and in the development of new medications.

The dataset provides comprehensive information about medications, including their substitutes, potential side effects, medical uses, chemical classification, habit-forming properties, therapeutic class, and action class. It is noteworthy that there are missing values in various columns, and a DtypeWarning is issued for columns (42, 43, 44, 45, 46, 47, 48) due to potentially mixed data types. Handling missing values and investigating the mixed data types are crucial steps in the preprocessing phase. The "Habit Forming" column is binary, indicating whether a medication is habit-forming or not. The "Therapeutic Class" column categorizes medications based on their therapeutic purposes. This dataset offers a rich source for analysis, allowing exploration of relationships between different attributes, classification tasks, and clustering based on medication characteristics. Figure 8.3a, b depicts the different habit-forming and therapeutic classes.

These graphs offer a comprehensive overview of medication development and usage, including potential risks and the need for careful management of side effects,

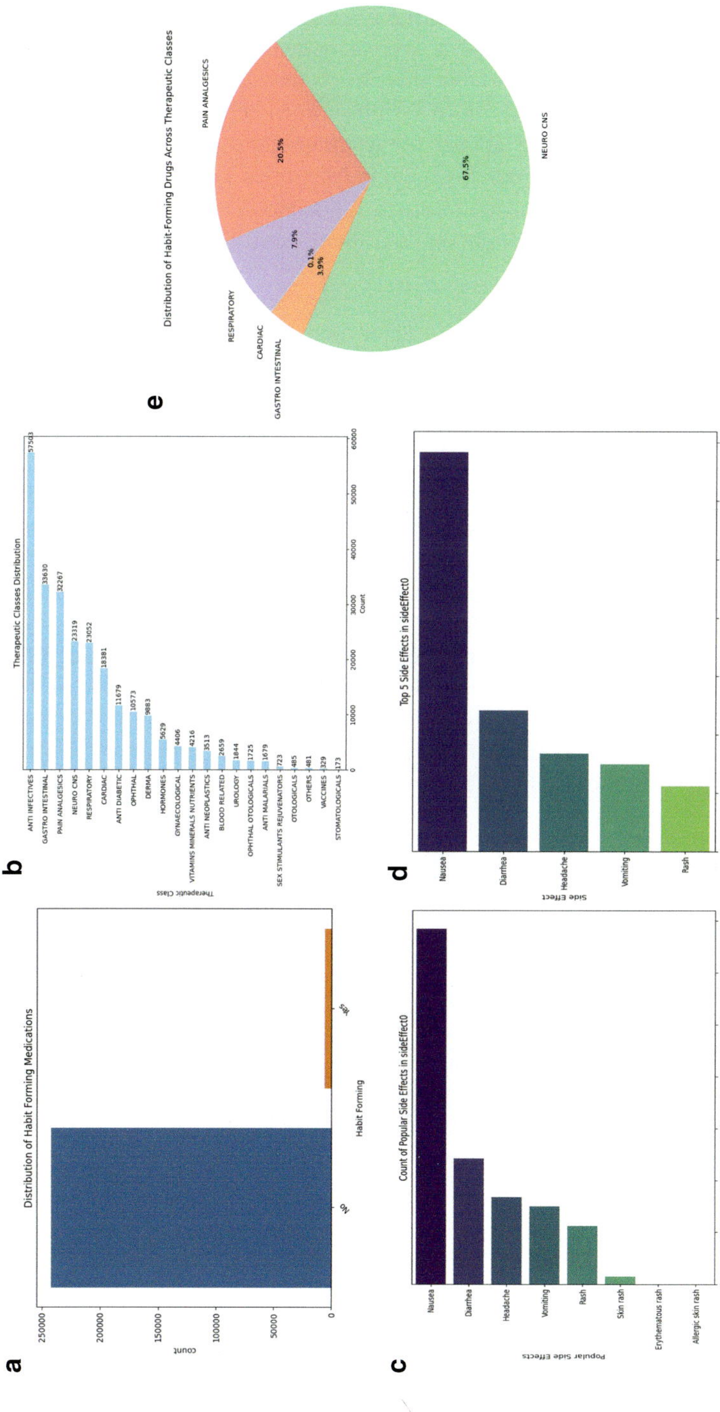

Fig. 8.3 (**a**) Distribution of habit-forming medications; (**b**) Therapeutic class distribution; (**c**) Total popular side effects in sideEffect0; (**d**) Top five side effects in sideeffect0; and (**e**) Distributions of farming drugs across therapeutic classes

particularly those that are most prevalent. The data could guide future research and healthcare practices, aiming to mitigate the risks associated with medication while addressing the therapeutic needs of a diverse patient population. Figure 8.3c, d depicts the total popularity and top five side effects in sideEffect0. Figure 8.3e presents an overview of the distribution of farming drugs across different therapeutic classes. The graphic depiction allows for a comprehensive examination of how drugs are allocated within various therapeutic categories in the context of farming practices. This visual representation offers insights into the prevalence and distribution patterns of drugs, shedding light on their therapeutic classes within the agricultural domain.

8.4.2 Analysis with Different Models

In Table 8.2 and Fig. 8.4, the evaluation of various machine learning models on the pharmacovigilance and pharmaceutical dataset, several key performance metrics were considered, including Accuracy and the Area Under the Receiver Operating Characteristic Curve (AUC). The Random Forest (RF) model emerged as the top-performing model with an accuracy of 97.62% and an AUC value of 0.7515. This indicates the model's robust ability to make accurate predictions and effectively distinguish between positive and negative classes in the dataset. K-Nearest Neighbors (KNN) demonstrated respectable performance with an accuracy of 95.22% and an AUC of 0.6875. Naive Bayes (NB) yielded an accuracy of 93.90% and an AUC of 0.6877, showcasing its reliability in classification tasks. Decision Tree (DT) achieved an accuracy of 89.76% and shared the highest AUC (0.7515) with RF. Support Vector Machine (SVM) exhibited an accuracy of 96.76%, though its AUC was relatively lower at 0.3776. The comprehensive evaluation underscores the Random Forest model's effectiveness in handling the pharmacovigilance and pharmaceutical dataset, making it a favorable choice for predictive modeling in this context.

Table 8.2 Comparison analysis of different models with performance metrics

S.No.	Model	Dataset	Accuracy	AUC
1	Random Forest (RF)	The pharmacovigilance and pharmaceutical dataset consists of 248,218 entries with 58 columns	0.9762	0.7515
2	K-Nearest Neighbors (KNN)		0.9522	0.6875
3	Naive Bayes (NB)		0.9390	0.6877
4	Decision Tree (DT)		0.8976	0.7515
5	Support Vector Machine (SVM)		0.9676	0.3776

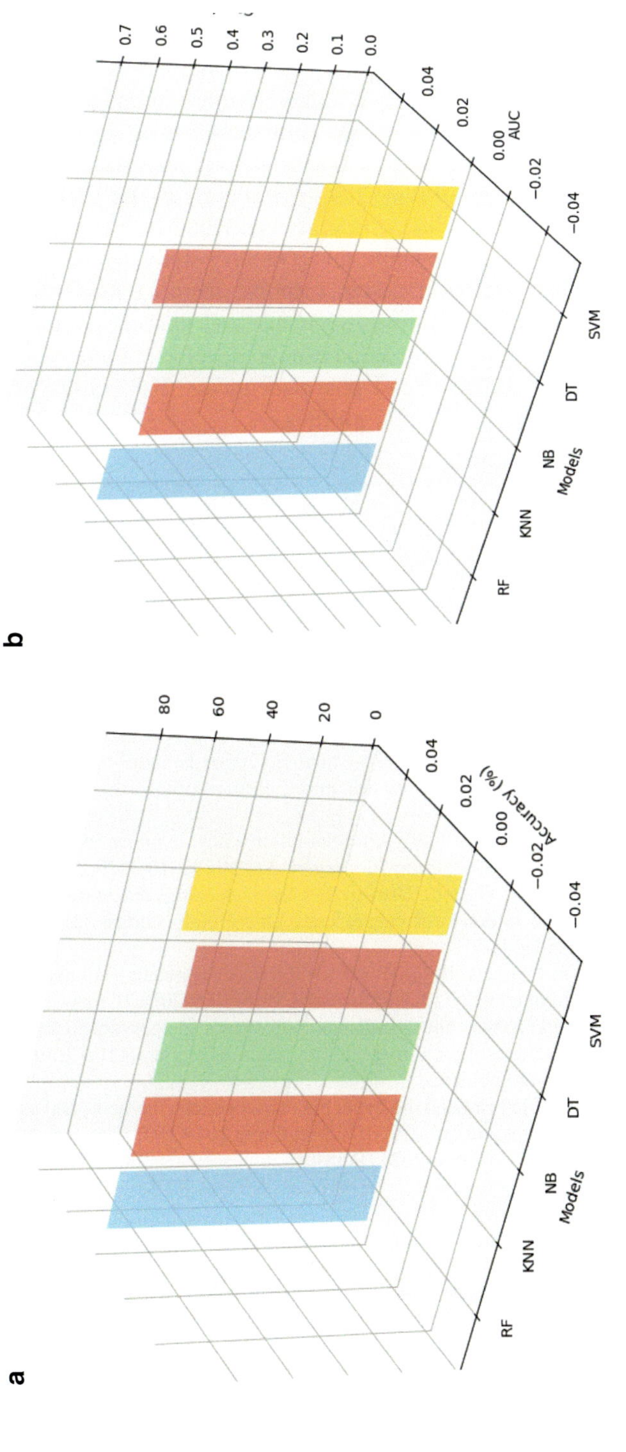

Fig. 8.4 Comparison of different machine learning models **(a)** Accuracy; and **(b)** AUC

8.5 Conclusion

A persistent issue in pharmacovigilance that is essential to patient safety is the timely and accurate establishment of safety profiles for pharmacovigilance and pharmaceuticals throughout their whole commercial lives. In this work, we proposed a high throughput model and method to identify pharmacovigilance and pharmaceutical safety signals by mining narrative reports in the EHR. By integrating NLP and statistical analysis with unstructured patient data, we have showcased the method's potential. As far as we know, this is the first study demonstrating the application of natural language processing, machine learning models, statistics, and unstructured patient data to pharmacovigilance and pharmaceutical datasets. The paradigm presented in this work may be used to develop automated, proactive, and prospective pharmacovigilance and pharmaceuticals that could swiftly identify novel adverse events and drug safety profiles.

References

Akay A, Dragomir A, Erlandsson B-E (2016) Assessing antidepressants using intelligent data monitoring and mining of online fora. IEEE J Biomed Health Inform 20:977–986. https://doi.org/10.1109/JBHI.2016.2539972

Almenoff JS, Pattishall EN, Gibbs TG et al (2007) Novel statistical tools for monitoring the safety of marketed drugs. Clin Pharmacol Ther 82:157–166. https://doi.org/10.1038/sj.clpt.6100258

Dai H-J, Wang C-K (2019) Classifying adverse drug reactions from imbalanced twitter data. Int J Med Inform 129:122–132. https://doi.org/10.1016/j.ijmedinf.2019.05.017

Dai H-J, Touray M, Jonnagaddala J, Syed-Abdul S (2016) Feature engineering for recognizing adverse drug reactions from twitter posts. Information 7:27. https://doi.org/10.3390/info7020027

De Oliveira AP, Tadeu Braga HF (2020) Artificial intelligence: learning and limitations. WSEAS Trans Adv Eng Educ 17:80–86. https://doi.org/10.37394/232010.2020.17.10

Dickerson SS, Boehmke M, Ogle C, Brown JK (2006) Seeking and managing hope: patients' experiences using the Internet for cancer care. Oncol Nurs Forum 33:E8–E17. https://doi.org/10.1188/06.ONF.E8-E17

European Commission: Brussels, Belgium (2020) Pharmacovigilance -Volume 2020. https://eur-lex.europa.eu/legal-content/EN/TXT/PDF/?uri=CELEX:52020DC0761

FDA (2009) ADRs: Prevalence and incidence. http://www.fda.gov/drugs/developmentapprovalprocess/developmentresources/druginteractionslabeling/ucm110632.htm\#ADRs:\%20Prevalence\%20and\%20Incidence

Gandomi A, Haider M (2015) Beyond the hype: big data concepts, methods, and analytics. Int J Inf Manag 35:137–144. https://doi.org/10.1016/j.ijinfomgt.2014.10.007

Ganesh P, Rawal BS, Peter A, Giri A (2021) POS-tagging based neural machine translation system for European languages using transformers. WSEAS Trans Inf Sci Appl 18:26–33. https://doi.org/10.37394/23209.2021.18.5

Gerber BS, Eiser AR (2001) The patient-physician relationship in the internet age: future prospects and the research agenda. J Med Internet Res 3:e15. https://doi.org/10.2196/jmir.3.2.e15

Gräßer F, Kallumadi S, Malberg H, Zaunseder S (2018) Aspect-based sentiment analysis of drug reviews applying cross-domain and cross-data learning. In: Proceedings of the 2018 international conference on digital health. ACM, Lyon, pp 121–125

Harpaz R, Haerian K, Chase HS, Friedman C (2010) Statistical mining of potential drug interaction adverse effects in FDA's spontaneous reporting system. AMIA Annu Symp Proc 2010:281–285

Hauben M, Bate A (2009) Decision support methods for the detection of adverse events in post-marketing data. Drug Discov Today 14:343–357. https://doi.org/10.1016/j.drudis.2008.12.012

Hochberg AM, Reisinger SJ, Pearson RK et al (2007) Using data mining to predict safety actions from FDA adverse event reporting system data. Drug Inform J 41:633–643. https://doi.org/10.1177/009286150704100510

Katragadda S, Karnati H, Pusala M et al (2015) Detecting adverse drug effects using link classification on twitter data. In: 2015 IEEE international conference on Bioinformatics and Biomedicine (BIBM). IEEE, Washington, DC, pp 675–679

Lazarou J, Pomeranz BH, Corey PN (1998) Incidence of adverse drug reactions in hospitalized patients: a meta-analysis of prospective studies. JAMA 279:1200. https://doi.org/10.1001/jama.279.15.1200

Lin W-S, Dai H-J, Jonnagaddala J et al (2015) Utilizing different word representation methods for twitter data in adverse drug reactions extraction. In: 2015 conference on Technologies and Applications of Artificial Intelligence (TAAI). IEEE, Tainan, pp 260–265

Mishra A, Malviya A, Aggarwal S (2015) Towards automatic pharmacovigilance: analysing patient reviews and sentiment on oncological drugs. In: 2015 IEEE International Conference on Data Mining Workshop (ICDMW). IEEE, Atlantic City, pp 1402–1409

Peters ME, Neumann M, Iyyer M et al (2018) Deep contextualized word representations. https://doi.org/10.48550/ARXIV.1802.05365

Sampathkumar H, Chen X, Luo B (2014) Mining adverse drug reactions from online healthcare forums using Hidden Markov Model. BMC Med Inform Decis Mak 14:91. https://doi.org/10.1186/1472-6947-14-91

Santoro A, Genov G, Spooner A et al (2017) Promoting and protecting public health: how the European Union pharmacovigilance system works. Drug Saf 40:855–869. https://doi.org/10.1007/s40264-017-0572-8

Sboev A, Selivanov A, Moloshnikov I et al (2022) Extraction of the relations among significant pharmacological entities in Russian-language reviews of Internet users on medications. BDCC 6:10. https://doi.org/10.3390/bdcc6010010

Schmider J, Kumar K, LaForest C et al (2019) Innovation in pharmacovigilance: use of artificial intelligence in adverse event case processing. Clin Pharma Ther 105:954–961. https://doi.org/10.1002/cpt.1255

Singh S, Thakur V, Tiwari V (2023) 250k Medicines usage, side effects and substitutes. In: Kaggle. https://www.kaggle.com/datasets/shudhanshusingh/250k-medicines-usage-side-effects-and-substitutes. Accessed 1 Oct 2024.

Tekin M, Etlioğlu M, Koyuncuoğlu Ö, Tekin E (2019) Data Mining in Digital Marketing. In: Durakbasa NM, Gencyilmaz MG (eds) Proceedings of the international symposium for production research 2018. Springer International Publishing, Cham, pp 44–61

Tyson TR (2000) The internet: tomorrow's portal to non-traditional health care services. J Ambul Care Manag 23:1–7. https://doi.org/10.1097/00004479-200004000-00002

Umefjord G, Petersson G, Hamberg K (2003) Reasons for consulting a doctor on the Internet: web survey of users of an ask the doctor service. J Med Internet Res 5:e26. https://doi.org/10.2196/jmir.5.4.e26

Wall J, Krummel T (2020) The digital surgeon: how big data, automation, and artificial intelligence will change surgical practice. J Pediatr Surg 55:47–50. https://doi.org/10.1016/j.jpedsurg.2019.09.008

World Health Organization (2017) World Health Organization. Pharmacovigilance. http://www.who.int/medicines/areas/quality_safety/safety_efficacy/pharmvigi/en/

Xu H, Van Durme B, Murray K (2021) BERT, mBERT, or BiBERT? A study on contextualized embeddings for neural machine translation. In: Proceedings of the 2021 conference on empirical methods in natural language processing. Association for Computational Linguistics, Online and Punta Cana, Dominican Republic, pp 6663–6675

Zucco C, Calabrese B, Cannataro M (2017) Sentiment analysis and affective computing for depression monitoring. In: 2017 IEEE international conference on Bioinformatics and Biomedicine (BIBM). IEEE, Kansas City, pp 1988–1995

Time Series Analysis in Reproductive Health Data

9

Priyanka Sharma, Tushar Gupta, Sudeepti Kulshrestha, Payal Gupta, Alakto Choudhury, Deepak Modi, and Abhishek Sengupta

Abstract

Reproductive health data is critical for identifying and focusing on reproductive health issues, developing effective policies and programs, and monitoring progress toward reproductive health goals. This book chapter delves into the integration of time series analysis methodologies through a discussion on the components of time series analysis data, discussing the trends of the data to determine if there is a factor that has been influencing the result of the data points. Further, it discusses the different types of data point variations such as seasonal variations, cyclical variations, and irregular variations. The chapter further focuses on the different types of time series models namely the additive and multiplicative models. For reproductive health, time series analysis is essential as it helps in the prediction of future results, the evaluation of previous performances, and the identification of underlying patterns and trends and has the potential to provide valuable insights into a variety of health data, including patient behavior and other factors that are reliant on the passage of time. The chapter also sheds light on the different types of reproductive health data on which time series analysis could be applied to and talks about the efficiency parameters of using time series analysis in reproductive health data.

P. Sharma (✉) · T. Gupta
Bioinformatics Technologies of India, Bareilly, India

S. Kulshrestha · P. Gupta · A. Choudhury · A. Sengupta
Systems Biology and Data Analytics Research Lab, Amity Institute of Biotechnology, Amity University, Uttar Pradesh, Noida, India

D. Modi
Molecular and Cellular Biology Laboratory, National Institute for Research in Reproductive and Child Health, Mumbai, India

A. Sengupta et al. (eds.), *Data-Driven Reproductive Health*,
https://doi.org/10.1007/978-981-97-7451-7_9

Keywords

Time series analysis · Reproductive health · Fertility rates · Maternal health Contraceptive rates

9.1 Introduction

Reproductive health data is essential for understanding and addressing reproductive health issues, developing effective policies and programs, and monitoring progress toward reproductive health goals. Key components of reproductive health data include fertility rates, contraceptive use, maternal health indicators, sexually transmitted infections (STIs), abortion rates, and adolescent reproductive health (Dixon-Mueller and Germain 2007). Time series analysis is a precise method of understanding and analyzing data points collected over a set period, recording them at consistent intervals over a set period. This helps in discovering patterns or similarities among data points and estimates variations over time.

For better consistency and reliability, data used in time series analysis must be highly curated and free of noise. Data must be preprocessed and filtered before analysis, ensuring essential data is included and highlighted, and any pattern or trend is not an outliner and may account for seasonal variance. For example, a survey of a metro line can be used to understand the occupancy patterns on different days of the week (Himeur et al. 2023). Time series analysis is a method used to analyze data from a series of time durations, which can be influenced by various factors such as social, natural, industrial, political, and economic factors (Brockwell 2010). The components of time series data can be categorized into secular/long-term trends, which are patterns followed by data points over a long period, and nonlinear trends, which are data points that do not follow a straight-line path. Seasonal variation refers to regular changes in data over a year, while cyclic variation involves recurrent ups and downs over a period. Irregular variation is the fluctuation of data points without any linkage or connection (Dagum and Laniel 1984). This method is used to decompose data into components, with two models: the additive and multiplicative models. The additive model represents data as a sum of four components, while the multiplicative model establishes a multiplicative relationship among these components. The deciding feature of time series analysis is its temporal dependence, meaning the distribution of an observation at a certain time point depends on the outcome of previous observations. Reproductive health data includes information about individuals' and populations' reproductive health, which is essential for understanding and addressing reproductive health concerns. Examples of data types, sources, and information related to reproductive health include family planning, mother and child health, sexually transmitted infections, and fertility (Htun et al. 2023).

This type of analysis helps analysts to estimate variations that occur in the data points collected from the same set of samples over a factor that in the case of time series is the 'TIME'. Time as a factor is a crucial variable because it indicates how the data adjusts throughout the data points as well as the finishing results (Ao and Fayek 2023). It gives us an additional source of information and helps to set the order of dependencies among the data points. Time series models can utilize the fact that observations closer together in time are closely related (Manickam et al. 2022).

To achieve greater consistency and dependability, the data that is utilized in time series analysis must consist of many data points that have been meticulously curated and are devoid of any kind of noise. This is because noise has the potential to interfere with the most important data points and to impede any association between points. The data must be preprocessed and filtered before the analysis to fulfill these criteria (Baidya and Jeong 2023). This will ensure that only the most important data is included and emphasized, while the noise and data that are not connected to the research are discarded. In addition to this, it is essential to make certain that any pattern or trend that is detected in the pattern is not an outliner and that it provides an explanation for seasonal variation.

9.1.1 Components of Time Series

The data that is the result of a succession of time durations may be analyzed with the assistance of time series analysis. Several elements might cause the data that is being acquired to be different. These aspects include social, natural, industrial, political, and economic factors. In the context of time series, these components are referred to as the components. One possible classification for the variance of the components of the time series data is as follows.

9.1.1.1 Secular/Long-Term Trend

A possible interpretation of this would be that the pattern that the data points are following. If the data points that are being gathered in the data are closely associated with a lack of variation and the points are seen following a set pattern over an extended period, this component is referred to as a Secular Trend or simply a Trend. A trend is observed in the data points if there is a factor that has been influencing the result of the data points for a considerable amount of time over a certain period. An example of this would be the rise in the birth rate of humans all over the world.

There are two types of trends being observed:

- Linear Trend:
- This type of trend is referred to as a linear trend, and it occurs when the data points in a time series analysis are closely associated with a continuous shift in the values. When this occurs, the points cluster around a straight line.
- Nonlinear Trend:
- This form of trend is referred to as a nonlinear trend, and it occurs when the data points do not have any specific link to each other, which causes them to seem different from one another. Additionally, they do not follow any path that is linear or clustered together.

9.1.1.2 Seasonal Variation

Seasonal variation is a sort of variation that occurs when the data points indicate regular changes in the data over a year. This type of variation is known as seasonal fluctuations (Koopman and Ooms 2006).

For example: the demand for sweaters decreases during the hot summer months, but the number of sweaters sold increases during the chilly winter months.

9.1.1.3 Cyclic Variation

This kind of variation is referred to as cyclic variation, and it occurs when the data goes through a series of increases and decreases throughout a length of time that is longer than a year.

Example: the valuation of stocks on the market?

9.1.1.4 Erratic/Irregular Variation

This refers to the fluctuation of data points in the time series analysis, in which each point appears to be independent of the others and there is no connectivity or relationship between them (Jebb et al. 2015). In terms of its occurrence, this kind of data is completely random. It is well known that this kind of data is comprised of irregular variation.

9.1.2 Models of Time Series Analysis

After understanding various components of the time series analysis, we need to focus on various models of time series analysis that help in the decomposition of the time series data into the mentioned components (Talaei-Khoei et al. 2019).

There are two models of time series analysis that help us to distinguish our data into components:

1. Additive model
2. Multiplicative model

9.1.2.1 Additive Model

In the additive model, the data is represented as a particular observation in a time series as the sum of these four components.

$$O = T + S + C + I$$

where 'O' represents the 'original data'; 'T' represents the 'trend'; 'S' represents the 'seasonal variations'; 'C' represents the 'cyclical variations'; and 'I' represents the 'irregular variations'.

In another way, we can write:

$$Y(t) = T(t) + S(t) + C(t) + I(t)$$

We use the additive model where neither the amplitude of the seasonal nor the amplitude of irregular variations changes with the level of the trend in the time series data.

9.1.2.2 Multiplicative Model

In this model, a multiplicative relationship is established among four components. So, the data is represented as a particular observation in a time series as the product of these four components:

$$O = T \times S \times C \times I$$

where '*O*' represents the 'original data'; '*T*' represents the 'trend'; '*S*' represents the 'seasonal variations'; '*C*' represents the 'cyclical variations'; and '*I*' represents the 'irregular variations'.

In another way, we can write:

$$Y(t) = T(t) \times S(t) \times C(t) \times I(t)$$

We use the multiplicative model where the amplitude of both the seasonal and irregular variations increase with the level of the trend in the time series data.

9.2 Methods of Time Series Analysis

For reproductive health, time series analysis is essential because it allows for the prediction of future results, the evaluation of previous performances, and the identification of underlying patterns and trends in a variety of time series analyses have the potential to provide valuable insights into a variety of health data, including patient behavior and other factors that are reliant on the passage of time. The field of reproductive health can make educated judgments, improve operations, and strengthen long-term strategy by utilizing these technological techniques (Lamaro Haintz et al. 2023).

As a result of the fact that various approaches serve diverse objectives and provide varying degrees of granularity and accuracy, health data need to understand the ways that are most suitable for their requirements.

9.2.1 Moving Average

It helps reduce the impact of long-term trends. Getting rid of noise and determining the overall direction in which values are going are two of its most useful applications.

9.2.2 Exponential Smoothing

This method is suitable for univariate data that contains a systematic trend or periodic component. Increased weight is given to recent observations, which enables modifications to be made more dynamically.

9.2.3 Autoregression

Utilizes previous observations as inputs for a regression equation to forecast future values. In situations when historical data is a reliable indicator, it is useful for making short-term forecasts.

9.2.4 Decomposition

The purpose of this is to improve both the understanding and the accuracy of forecasts by breaking down a time series into its fundamental components, which are trend, seasonality, and residuals.

9.2.5 Time Series Clustering

To assist in the identification of archetypes or patterns in sequential data, an unsupervised approach is utilized to classify data points according to their similarities.

9.2.6 Wavelet Analysis

This method is effective for analyzing time series data that is not steady. It assists in the identification of patterns across a variety of scales, or the resolution of data points based on similarity, hence assisting in the identification of archetypes or trends in sequential data collection.

9.2.7 Intervention Analysis

Evaluate the influence that external occurrences have on a time series, such as the impact of a change in policy or the impact of a marketing campaign.

9.2.8 Box-Jenkins ARIMA Models

This approach models time series data by concentrating on the utilization of previous behavior and mistakes. It is assumed that the data may be described by a linear function of its average values in the past.

9.2.9 Box-Jenkins Multivariate Models

Just like ARIMA, however, it takes into consideration several different factors. When additional factors affect a single time series, this is useful.

9.2.10 Holt-Winters Exponential Smoothing

The most suitable for data that has a clear trend and seasonality. Weighted averages are incorporated, and the formulae for exponential smoothing are expanded upon throughout the process.

9.3 Reproductive Health Data (Types, Sources, Information)

Information about the reproductive health of individuals and populations is included in the scope of reproductive health data, which comprises a wide variety of information. It is essential to have this information to comprehend and address a variety of reproductive health concerns, including but not limited to family planning, mother and child health, sexually transmitted infections (STIs), fertility, and other related topics (Götmark and Andersson 2020). An overview of the many types of data, sources of data, and information connected to reproductive health is presented here.

9.3.1 Types of Reproductive Health Data

9.3.1.1 Fertility Data

Comprises data about the number of births, fertility rates, and patterns in family planning. This data is crucial for evaluating population growth and determining the success of family planning programs (Tapales et al. 2019).

9.3.1.2 Maternal Health Data

Concentrates on the well-being of expectant mothers, encompassing factors such as antenatal care, maternal mortality rates, and difficulties during pregnancy and delivery (Tapales et al. 2019).

9.3.1.3 Contraceptive Use Data

Offers valuable information on the frequency and varieties of contraception techniques employed by individuals and populations. This data is crucial for family planning activities (Tapales et al. 2019).

9.3.1.4 Sexual Health Data

Includes information on sexually transmitted diseases (STIs), prevalence of HIV/AIDS, and trends of sexual behavior. This information is beneficial for developing preventative and awareness initiatives (Tapales et al. 2019).

9.3.1.5 Infertility Data

Contains data about the prevalence of infertility, the factors contributing to infertility, and the utilization of assisted reproductive technologies (ART) such as in vitro fertilization (IVF) (Tapales et al. 2019).

9.3.1.6 Abortion Data

Contains information about the frequency of abortions, the techniques employed, and the level of safety associated with abortion procedures. This information is crucial for the development of reproductive health policies and the improvement of maternity care (Tapales et al. 2019).

9.3.1.7 Adolescent Reproductive Health Data

Concentrates on the reproductive health of teenagers, encompassing topics such as early pregnancies, availability of sexual education, and reproductive healthcare services for youth (Tapales et al. 2019).

9.3.2 Sources of Reproductive Health Data

There are different sources of reproductive health data, some of them are below (Rousseau 2023).

9.3.2.1 Healthcare Facilities

Hospitals, clinics, and healthcare centers offer information on prenatal treatment, childbirth, and mother health results.

9.3.2.2 Public Surveys and Censuses

Surveys and censuses are conducted at a national level to gather information on reproduction rates, contraceptive usage, and other variables related to reproductive health.

9.3.2.3 Health Records and Registers

Electronic health records and population registers save essential data about births, deaths, and numerous reproductive health occurrences.

9.3.2.4 Public Health Agencies

National and international health agencies gather and distribute reproductive health statistics derived from many sources.

9.3.2.5 Research Studies

Scientific studies and research initiatives enhance our understanding of certain facets of reproductive health, such as the effects of particular therapies or patterns in reproductive behaviors.

9.3.2.6 NGOs

Nongovernmental organizations (NGOs) engaged in the field of reproductive health frequently gather and analyze data to assess the efficacy of their programs and lobby for alterations in policies.

9.3.3 Information Provided by Reproductive Health Data

9.3.3.1 Demographic Trends

Encompass several factors such as population growth rates, age-specific fertility rates, and demographic transitions (Zhang et al. 2022).

9.3.3.2 Health Outcomes

Rates of maternal mortality, rates of newborn mortality, and other health indicators associated with reproductive events.

9.3.3.3 Access to Healthcare Services

Provision of comprehensive and easily obtainable reproductive healthcare services, encompassing family planning and maternity care.

9.3.3.4 Behavioral Patterns

Information regarding sexual behaviors, patterns of contraceptive usage, and trends in choices related to family planning.

9.3.3.5 Epidemiological Insights

Prevalence and occurrence rates of sexually transmitted infections (STIs), HIV/AIDS, and other disorders connected to reproductive health.

9.3.3.6 Policy Impact Assessment

Data is utilized to evaluate the effects of reproductive health policies and programs, guiding policymakers in making decisions that are supported by empirical evidence.

9.3.3.7 Social and Economic Implications

Analyzing the impact of socioeconomic factors, such as education and income levels, on reproductive health outcomes.

9.4 Use of Time Series Analysis in Reproductive Health Data Analysis

The field of reproductive health data is now being investigated through a variety of research investigations, and time series analysis is being utilized to ascertain the outcomes and draw conclusions. The research that Zhang and his colleagues conducted and published in their paper titled "The Prediction of Preterm Birth Using Time-Series Technology-Based Machine Learning: Retrospective Cohort Study" is an example of such a publication. This study investigated and evaluated the risk of preterm delivery in 5187 pregnant Chinese women by using data from obstetric electronic medical records (EMR). The long short-term memory (LSTM) machine learning model, which operates on the concept of time-series technology, was built and utilized by the researchers to analyze the predicted and recurring obstetric examination records that occurred during pregnancy. This was done to train the preterm birth screening model. This model exhibited better and more promising outcomes when compared to standard cross-sectional research. The model had an accuracy of about 0.739, a sensitivity of 0.407, a specificity of 0.982, and an area under the curve (AUC) of 0.651. Additionally, the findings of this study indicate that parameters such as blood pressure, lipids, blood glucose, and uric acid all have a significant impact on the occurrence of premature delivery (Oomman and Ganatra 2002).

9.5 Efficiency of Using Time Series Analysis in Reproductive Health Data (Application, Advantages, Uniqueness)

When applied to data about reproductive health, time series analysis turns out to be a very effective and advantageous method. The application of time series analysis in the field of reproductive health comes with several distinct advantages and characteristics, including the following.

9.5.1 Identification of Temporal Trends

Using time series analysis, it is possible to recognize patterns and trends in reproductive health indicators over a period. These indicators include changes in fertility rates, maternal death rates, and the use of contraceptives. When politicians and healthcare professionals have a better understanding of temporal patterns, they are better able to evaluate the efficacy of treatments and more efficiently distribute resources (Wiemken et al. 2023).

9.5.2 Seasonal Patterns and Variability

It is possible to uncover seasonal patterns in reproductive health outcomes through the use of time series analysis. These variations might include the timing of births or fluctuations in the incidence of illnesses. The recognition of seasonal trends is essential for the design of focused treatments during periods of the year and for the adaptation of healthcare services following these patterns (Zhou et al. 2018).

9.5.3 Forecasting Future Trends

The application of time series models allows for the prediction of future reproductive health outcomes, which is beneficial for both the planning of resources and the formulation of policies (Kruk et al. 2018). Healthcare systems can predict the demand for services, allocate resources, and put preventative measures into effect in a timely way if they have performed accurate forecasting.

9.5.4 Monitoring and Evaluation of Interventions

The use of time series analysis makes it possible to evaluate the effects of reproductive health policies and interventions throughout certain periods. It gives insights into the success of programs, which enables modifications and improvements to be made based on patterns that have been noticed in health indicators (Li et al. 2022).

9.5.5 Data-Driven Decision-Making

Using time series analysis, decision-makers can make decisions that are informed and driven by data about the allocation of resources, the design of policies, and the development of programs. Those in charge of making decisions can prioritize interventions and distribute resources to the areas that require them the most when they depend on past data trends (Starbird et al. 2016).

9.5.6 Understanding Long-Term Patterns

Long-term changes in reproductive health can be uncovered with time series analysis. These changes may include adjustments in family planning methods or advances in the utilization of maternal healthcare. For establishing policies and programs that are sustainable and that address the ever-changing requirements of reproductive health, this understanding is crucial (Lince-Deroche et al. 2020).

9.5.7 Early Detection of Anomalies or Emergencies

One way to find sudden spikes or abnormalities in reproductive health indicators is using time series analysis. For example, unexpected rises in maternal death can be identified by this method. The ability to recognize health problems at an early stage enables rapid reactions, emergency interventions, and the prevention of future escalation of health problems (Whitmill et al. 2016).

9.5.8 Tailored Interventions and Targeted Outreach

The examination of time series can assist in the identification of subpopulations or geographic areas that have reproductive health requirements. This information makes it possible to build focused interventions and outreach programs to address the specific difficulties that are encountered by various groups (Midboe et al. 2020).

9.5.9 Integration with Other Data Sources

The use of time series analysis in conjunction with other data sources, such as socio-economic indicators, can result in a more thorough knowledge of the patterns in reproductive health. When it comes to addressing the myriad of factors that have an impact on reproductive health outcomes, integrated analyses are a significant contributor to a holistic approach (Midboe et al. 2020).

9.6 Future Directions

The routes that time series analysis in reproductive health data will take in the future offer a great deal of promise for its potential to revolutionize healthcare practices and improve outcomes for both individuals and communities. One of the most important approaches is the incorporation of multi-modal data, which involves the combination of time series information with genetic, demographic, and environmental data to provide a comprehensive knowledge of the variables that influence reproductive health. Taking such a broad approach makes it possible to conduct a more nuanced study, which reveals complicated patterns and interdependencies that may be essential for the development of personalized treatment plans. The landscape is constantly shifting, and machine learning and predictive modeling are positioned to play a significant part in this transformation. There is a wide range of reproductive health outcomes that may be predicted using sophisticated models. These outcomes include fertility patterns, pregnancy risks, and the forecasting of wider trends in reproductive health. By enabling proactive and individualized therapies that are based on expected trajectories and risk assessments, the deployment of these models has the potential to revolutionize the healthcare industry. When it comes to the future of time series analysis in reproductive health, real-time monitoring and intervention options represent yet another frontier. The use of technologies that can detect abnormalities or trends in real-time enables healthcare practitioners to respond swiftly, which has the potential to prevent problems and improve patient outcomes. By enabling continuous data collection, mobile health (mHealth) apps further enhance this potential. These applications include the tracking of menstrual cycles and the monitoring of hormone levels, and they provide a rich stream of information that can be analyzed. Collaboration between data scientists and experts working in the healthcare industry is necessary. To guarantee that the insights generated from time series analysis are properly translated into medical practice, it is necessary to bridge the gap between scientific breakthroughs and clinical relevance. The incorporation of global health views into research endeavors is also recommended, to recognize the myriad of cultural, social, and geographical factors that have an impact on reproductive health outcomes on a worldwide scale. Taking use of the potential of time series analysis to improve patient outcomes, increase personalized treatment, and contribute to a more comprehensive knowledge of reproductive health, these collective prospects represent a paradigm change in the field of reproductive healthcare.

9.7 Conclusion

In summary, time series analysis in reproductive health data has the potential to revolutionize healthcare practices and outcomes. It allows for in-depth insights into trends, patterns, and predictive modeling, leading to a better understanding of reproductive health dynamics. The integration of multi-modal data, advanced machine learning models, and real-time monitoring systems can personalize interventions and optimize healthcare strategies. Longitudinal studies and cohort analysis contribute to a nuanced comprehension of reproductive health over extended periods. Ethical considerations and data privacy are important for responsible research practices. Collaboration between data scientists and healthcare professionals is crucial to effectively translate insights into clinical applications. A global perspective acknowledges the diverse factors influencing reproductive health outcomes. Explainable AI reinforces the credibility and interpretability of results, building trust among healthcare professionals and patients. Ethical collection and responsible use of reproductive health data, along with technological advancements, will continue to shape healthcare delivery. Time series analysis can improve individual patient care and inform public health policies, advancing reproductive health globally. Embracing future directions and emerging technologies will promote reproductive well-being and empower individuals to make informed choices about their reproductive health.

Acknowledgments The authors would like to acknowledge the use of AI-based tools such as Quillbot and Grammarly to improve readability and summarize some parts of the text. The authors have further reviewed the text and take full responsibility for the text.

References

Ao S-I, Fayek H (2023) Continual deep learning for time series modeling. Sensors 23:7167. https://doi.org/10.3390/s23167167

Baidya R, Jeong H (2023) Anomaly detection in time series data using reversible instance normalized anomaly transformer. Sensors 23:9272. https://doi.org/10.3390/s23229272

Brockwell PJ (2010) Time series analysis. In: International encyclopedia of education. Elsevier, pp 474–481

Dagum EB, Laniel NJD (1984) [Issues involved with the seasonal adjustment of economic time series]: comment. J Bus Econ Stat 2:328. https://doi.org/10.2307/1391270

Dixon-Mueller R, Germain A (2007) Fertility regulation and reproductive health in the millennium development goals: the search for a perfect indicator. Am J Public Health 97:45–51. https://doi.org/10.2105/AJPH.2005.068056

Götmark F, Andersson M (2020) Human fertility in relation to education, economy, religion, contraception, and family planning programs. BMC Public Health 20:265. https://doi.org/10.1186/s12889-020-8331-7

Himeur Y, Elnour M, Fadli F et al (2023) AI-big data analytics for building automation and management systems: a survey, actual challenges and future perspectives. Artif Intell Rev 56:4929–5021. https://doi.org/10.1007/s10462-022-10286-2

Htun HH, Biehl M, Petkov N (2023) Survey of feature selection and extraction techniques for stock market prediction. Financ Innov 9:26. https://doi.org/10.1186/s40854-022-00441-7

Jebb AT, Tay L, Wang W, Huang Q (2015) Time series analysis for psychological research: examining and forecasting change. Front Psychol 6. https://doi.org/10.3389/fpsyg.2015.00727
Koopman SJ, Ooms M (2006) Forecasting daily time series using periodic unobserved components time series models. Comput Stat Data Anal 51:885–903. https://doi.org/10.1016/j.csda.2005.09.009
Kruk ME, Gage AD, Arsenault C et al (2018) High-quality health systems in the Sustainable Development Goals era: time for a revolution. Lancet Glob Health 6:e1196–e1252. https://doi.org/10.1016/S2214-109X(18)30386-3
Lamaro Haintz G, Hanna L, Taket A (2023) Understanding community engagement in sexual and reproductive health and rights promotion in the Eastern Cape, South Africa: a conceptual framework to inform practice. Health Soc Care Community 2023:1–10. https://doi.org/10.1155/2023/6662437
Li C, Chen Y, Shang Y (2022) A review of industrial big data for decision making in intelligent manufacturing. Eng Sci Technol Int J 29:101021. https://doi.org/10.1016/j.jestch.2021.06.001
Lince-Deroche N, Sully EA, Firestein L, Riley T (2020) Budgeting for comprehensive sexual and reproductive health and rights under universal health coverage. Sex Reprod Health Matters 28:1779631. https://doi.org/10.1080/26410397.2020.1779631
Manickam P, Mariappan SA, Murugesan SM et al (2022) Artificial Intelligence (AI) and Internet of Medical Things (IoMT) assisted biomedical systems for intelligent healthcare. Biosensors 12:562. https://doi.org/10.3390/bios12080562
Midboe AM, Gray C, Cheng H et al (2020) Implementation of health-focused interventions in vulnerable populations: protocol for a scoping review. BMJ Open 10:e036937. https://doi.org/10.1136/bmjopen-2020-036937
Oomman N, Ganatra BR (2002) Sex selection: the systematic elimination of girls. Reprod Health Matters 10:184–188. https://doi.org/10.1016/S0968-8080(02)00029-0
Rousseau C (2023) Climate change and sexual and reproductive health: what implications for future research? Sex Reprod Health Matters 31:2232196. https://doi.org/10.1080/26410397.2023.2232196
Starbird E, Norton M, Marcus R (2016) Investing in family planning: key to achieving the sustainable development goals. Glob Health Sci Pract 4:191–210. https://doi.org/10.9745/GHSP-D-15-00374
Talaei-Khoei A, Wilson JM, Kazemi S-F (2019) Period of measurement in time-series predictions of disease counts from 2007 to 2017 in Northern Nevada: analytics experiment. JMIR Public Health Surveill 5:e11357. https://doi.org/10.2196/11357
Tapales A, Desai S, Leong E (2019) Data opportunities for studying the sexual and reproductive health of immigrants in the United States. J Health Care Poor Underserved 30:560–586. https://doi.org/10.1353/hpu.2019.0031
Whitmill J, Blanton C, Doraiswamy S et al (2016) Retrospective analysis of reproductive health indicators in the United Nations High Commissioner for Refugees post-emergency camps 2007–2013. Confl Heal 10:3. https://doi.org/10.1186/s13031-016-0069-6
Wiemken TL, Khan F, Puzniak L et al (2023) Seasonal trends in COVID-19 cases, hospitalizations, and mortality in the United States and Europe. Sci Rep 13:3886. https://doi.org/10.1038/s41598-023-31057-1
Zhang Y, Lu S, Wu Y et al (2022) The prediction of preterm birth using time-series technology-based machine learning: retrospective cohort study. JMIR Med Inform 10:e33835. https://doi.org/10.2196/33835
Zhou L, Zhao P, Wu D et al (2018) Time series model for forecasting the number of new admission inpatients. BMC Med Inform Decis Mak 18:39. https://doi.org/10.1186/s12911-018-0616-8

Data Mining Ethics in Reproductive Health

10

Anukriti Saran, Chhavi Rawat, Shreeya Singh, and Saumya Pandey

Abstract

Data mining is a powerful tool for analyzing large datasets, particularly in the field of reproductive health, enabling the identification of patterns and the extraction of valuable insights. It aids in problem-solving, trend prediction, risk minimization, and the discovery of new opportunities for patient care. This chapter discusses the different methodologies for ethical data mining in reproductive health. It focuses on the importance of identifying the purpose and scope of the data before the extraction of data and also emphasizes the importance of informed consent and privacy and confidentiality to identify vulnerabilities in the system or to detect suspicious activities. The chapter further focusses on the transparent data practices that are fundamental in ethical data management, ensuring openness and accountability throughout the data lifecycle. It also explores relevant rules and guidelines, presenting a holistic view of the evolving ethical standards. We will examine the specific regulations and guidelines applicable to this field, helping readers grasp the changing ethical landscape. Real-world case studies will illustrate our insights, shedding light on the ethical implications that arise from the convergence of data mining and reproductive health. Ultimately, this chapter contributes to a deeper understanding of the ethical dimensions guiding data mining practices in this critical healthcare field.

Keywords

Data mining · Reproductive health · Ethical considerations · Data privacy Ethical approaches · Guidelines · Healthcare decision-making

A. Saran (✉) · C. Rawat · S. Singh · S. Pandey
Department of Bioscience & Biotechnology, Banasthali Vidyapith, Tonk, Rajasthan, India

A. Sengupta et al. (eds.), *Data-Driven Reproductive Health*,
https://doi.org/10.1007/978-981-97-7451-7_10

10.1 Introduction

Ethical data mining in reproductive health requires a responsible, transparent, fair, and unbiased collection of data and its analysis and use related to reproductive afflictions. Ensuring ethical data mining rules can ensure that the privacy and confidentiality of the individual can be protected throughout the data mining process.

Delving into the ethical considerations, this chapter scrutinizes the challenges posed by data privacy and security in the context of reproductive health. It underscores the paramount importance of safeguarding sensitive information and discusses the ethical approaches taken to navigate the complexities of obtaining permissions for data collection and analysis.

10.2 Methodology for Ethical Data Mining in Reproductive Health

For the ethical data mining process for data on reproductive health issues, the methods are outlined below.

10.2.1 Purpose and Scope of the Data

Before the start of the mining process, it is crucial to clearly express the aims and objectives of the project in reproductive health. The purpose and scope of the data mining project provide a foundation for making the process transparent and fair.

By defining the scope of the project, the type of data to be collected for some specific reproductive health problem can be specified. This makes the process of collection of data less cumbersome. It also ensures that the data collected is not redundant and only meaningful data is collected from which it will be easy to explore datasets to identify patterns and extract valuable insights using statistical, machine learning, and database techniques (Feeley et al. 2020).

10.2.2 Informed Consent

During the collection of data, it is essential to inform the individual of the specific boundaries of data usage, mitigating the risk of misuse of the data or some other unintended repercussions. The individual should be informed of why their data related to reproductive health is collected and used, and it should be ensured that the individual willingly and knowingly agrees to the collection and use of the data (Dunn 2001).

10.2.3 Privacy and Confidentiality

According to the Digital Personal Data Protection Act, 2023, to guarantee the privacy of the individual's data, strong protection measures should be implemented. Some keys to data protection could be as follows:

- Encrypting data during its transmission over networks and storage.
- Strict access control should be implemented and provided to authorized personnel.
- Anonymization techniques (for example randomization, pseudonymization, K-anonymity, etc.) can be implemented to remove personally identifiable information (PII) from the data.
- Minimum data, necessary only for the project, should be collected and retained. Avoid collection of sensitive information that is not necessary for the project.
- The data should be stored on secured and certified storage devices and transmitted over channels using secure protocols, to prevent unauthorized access.
- Personnel handling the data should be made aware of and trained on data privacy and security protocols.
- For the events of a breach of data, a detailed response plan should be made which includes communication protocols, notification procedures, and steps to mitigate the impact of the breach.
- For the protection of reproductive health data, understanding legal requirements is essential, and it should be ensured that the practices align with the requirements.
- The data should be securely and irreversibly deleted from all storage devices.
- When working with third-party vendors, assess their data protection protocols and ensure they maintain the same high standards for protecting reproductive health data.
- Custom software or applications' data mining process should incorporate secure coding practices to avoid vulnerabilities that can be exploited by attackers.
- Regular security monitoring should be conducted to identify vulnerabilities in the system or to detect suspicious activities.

10.2.4 Data Quality

Data quality is the measure of the condition of data based on it being complete, accurate, consistent, reliable, and up to date. It is critical to ensure the quality of data to make informed decisions and draw meaningful insights.

In reproductive health care issues, in getting quality data certain issues are faced, incomplete data, duplicate data or outdated information, and more. To resolve these issues, a multifaceted approach is required which consists of data profiling, data auditing, data validation and cleansing, comparing data from multiple sources, monitoring data quality metrics, user feedback, and domain expert involvement. By implementing these strategies the user may point the issues relating to the data and it helps to make accurate and reliable decisions (Cossio-Gil et al. 2022).

10.2.5 Transparent Data Practices

Transparent data practices are fundamental in ethical data management, ensuring openness and accountability throughout the data lifecycle. This involves clearly articulating the purpose and scope of data collection, processing, and analysis, fostering understanding among stakeholders. Transparency extends to methodologies and algorithms used, elucidating the steps taken in deriving insights. Providing information on data sources, processing steps, and any potential biases contributes to a more comprehensible and trustworthy data ecosystem. Open communication about findings, limitations, and potential impacts helps stakeholders make informed decisions. In summary, transparent data practices involve clear and accessible documentation of every stage in the data process, fostering trust and ethical conduct in data-driven endeavors (Porter and Lee 2013; Leusder et al. 2023; Etges et al. 2020).

10.2.6 Fair and Unbiased Algorithm

Certain algorithms may exhibit biases towards specific features, potentially resulting in the underfitting of data and incomplete representation of the entire dataset. It is imperative to assess and mitigate these biases in algorithms to ensure equitable representation across diverse demographic groups. Regular monitoring and updates to the algorithm are essential to address emerging biases and maintain a commitment to fair and unbiased data analysis over time (Aktar et al. 2022).

10.2.7 Data Governance and Compliance

A paramount aspect of ethical data mining involves clearly defining data ownership and control mechanisms, thereby empowering individuals with agency over decisions about their data. This encompasses transparent communication of how their information will be used and shared. Additionally, it is imperative to establish a system that allows individuals the flexibility to modify or withdraw their consent at any stage of the data mining process. This ensures that individuals maintain control over their personal information and can make informed choices regarding its utilization, reinforcing the principles of privacy and autonomy in the realm of data mining.

10.2.8 Data Ownership and Control

Establishing robust data ownership and control mechanisms is pivotal to endowing individuals with the authority to make informed decisions about their data. It is imperative to articulate clear guidelines delineating the ownership structure and how control over data will be exercised. Moreover, in adherence to ethical principles, it is essential to offer individuals the flexibility to modify or withdraw their consent at any juncture throughout the data mining process. This commitment not only aligns with privacy standards but also reinforces a culture of transparency and respect for individuals' autonomy in the context of data management (Aktar et al. 2022).

10.2.9 Monitoring and Auditing

In ethical data mining, the implementation of rigorous monitoring and auditing processes is paramount. This proactive approach involves continuous scrutiny to ensure strict adherence to established ethical guidelines throughout the entire data mining lifecycle. By subjecting data mining practices to regular and systematic reviews, organizations can identify potential ethical concerns, assess the effectiveness of existing protocols, and promptly address emerging issues. This commitment to ongoing monitoring and auditing not only enhances transparency but also underscores dedication to upholding ethical standards, fostering trust among stakeholders, and promoting responsible data management practices in an ever-evolving landscape.

10.2.10 Collaboration and Stakeholders

To ensure a collaborative and ethical approach to data mining in healthcare, active engagement with key stakeholders is essential. This includes fostering partnerships with healthcare professionals, researchers, and the broader community. By involving these stakeholders from the outset, a more comprehensive understanding of ethical considerations can be gained, and diverse perspectives can be incorporated into the data mining process. Furthermore, soliciting continuous feedback from these stakeholders becomes integral to refining and enhancing the ethical framework over time. This iterative feedback loop not only strengthens the ethical foundation of data mining practices but also establishes a dynamic and responsive framework that aligns with the evolving needs and concerns of the healthcare ecosystem (Porter and Lee 2013; Leusder et al. 2023; Etges et al. 2020).

10.2.11 Public Communication

In the context of ethical data mining in reproductive health, transparent and responsible public communication is imperative. It involves articulating findings, methodologies, and implications in a clear and accessible manner, avoiding sensationalism or misrepresentation. By disseminating information responsibly, the aim is to foster understanding among the public, healthcare professionals, and relevant stakeholders. This communication strategy not only upholds ethical principles but also contributes to building trust. It emphasizes the positive impact of the data mining research on reproductive health outcomes while respecting privacy and confidentiality. A commitment to ethical public communication ensures that the broader community remains informed, engaged, and supportive of advancements in reproductive health research derived from ethical data mining practices (Dunn 2001).

10.3 Appropriateness, Bias, and Fairness in the Application of Machine Learning in Health Contexts

Appropriateness emphasizes the importance of aligning machine learning algorithms with specific contexts and populations, considering the implications of automated decision-making in critical scenarios. The example of a pneumonia prediction algorithm highlights the significance of framing appropriate questions and involving domain experts in algorithm design (Baik et al. 2023).

Addressing unbalanced data is crucial, particularly in global health applications. The paper suggests methods like resampling, ensemble methods, and hyperparameter tuning to mitigate the impact of imbalanced datasets. It emphasizes the need to adapt models to specific populations to avoid misclassification errors (Banerjee et al. 2019).

Bias in algorithms is a systematic error or tendency to favor one outcome over another. It can result from human-designed machine learning algorithms and flawed training data. Bias can be implicit or explicit, arising from data sampling issues, algorithmic idiosyncrasies, equipment design, or unforeseen correlations in the data. Sampling bias is common, caused by unbalanced or missing training data, while implicit bias stems from unforeseen variable correlations (Dawn et al. 2008). Algorithmic bias is separate from ethics and is a mathematical consequence. Fairness is determined by ethical or legal principles, and bias evaluation is essential for adjusting machine learning models to meet fairness constraints (Bognar 2015). Facial detection algorithms showed significant bias against dark-skinned women, revealing issues with image features in the algorithm. Passport application algorithms rejected Asian applicants due to bias in processing facial images from different ethnic groups. Bias mitigation involves examining and adjusting processing algorithms, addressing bias at the data collection stage, and using regularization constraints or adversarial learning in prediction algorithms. Testing for bias at all stages of algorithm development is crucial, even with emerging mitigation methods (Davies 2023; Prunty et al. 2023).

Fairness in machine learning models is assessed against legal or ethical principles, varying across governments and cultures. Applications like diagnostic prediction, admissions decisions, and insurance premium calculations in healthcare can lead to unfair outcomes. Fairness can be evaluated at the individual or group level. Individual fairness aims for customized treatment based on similar characteristics, while group fairness considers demographic groups defined by race, gender, or socioeconomic status. Fairness criteria are often applied to binary classifiers with positive and negative outcomes. Fairness can be measured through equal outcomes, equality of opportunity, or equality of odds, each addressing different aspects of decision-making. The choice of fairness definition depends on local circumstances,

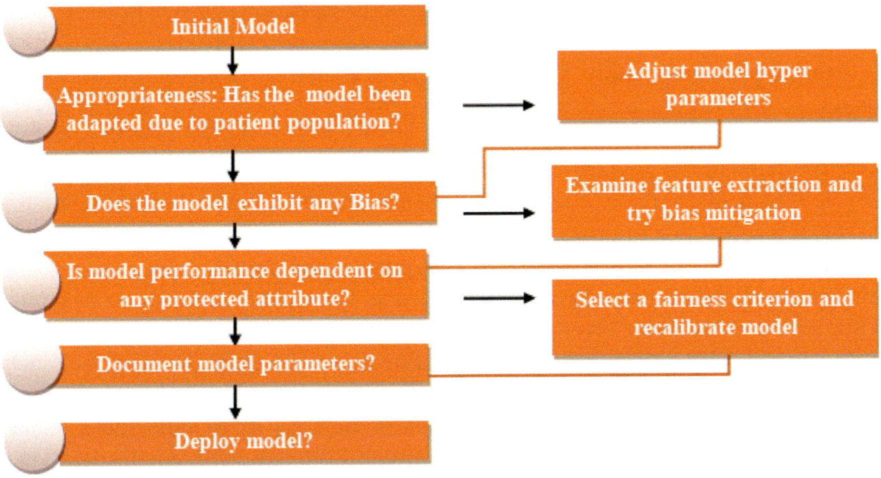

Fig. 10.1 Workflow diagram showing steps required to examine a model for bias, fairness, and appropriate use before deployment

applicable legal principles, and ethical considerations (Dot et al. 2020; Prunty et al. 2023; Bindemann and Burton 2009).

Some legal mandates may enforce specific fairness criteria, necessitating compliance. The acceptance of machine learning models in healthcare depends on factors like fairness. Future use may require disclosure from developers regarding the model's validity conditions and situations where it should not be used (Chua et al. 2022; Rajkomar et al. 2018). Regulatory frameworks for algorithms in medicine are currently undeveloped. Steps required to examine a model for bias, fairness, and appropriate use before deployment have been illustrated in Fig. 10.1. A workflow diagram is suggested for researchers in global health, emphasizing additional analysis and tuning before deploying machine learning models. Key considerations include fairness, stakeholder involvement, and disclosure of model limitations and validity.

10.4 Ethical Consideration

Health now involves overall well-being, fitness, and mental stability, with the body's protection tied to self-preservation. Autonomy is crucial, giving individuals the right to choose about their bodies and data, protected by medical confidentiality. Traditional medical data confidentiality faces challenges due to technology, data matching, and mining, raising ethical issues. Data techniques like matching and mining are used in healthcare, posing privacy concerns for patient information. Sensing technologies in healthcare heighten worries about patient privacy. Technology, healthcare data use, and handling sensitive information increase patient concerns about medical privacy. Data mining and profiling raise ethical issues, highlighting the need for ethical management of medical data (Chen et al. 2021; Pika et al. 2020).

Ethical principles apply to various aspects of human activity, encompassing interactions in healthcare, commerce, employment, and politics, as well as interactions with animals and the environment. In the healthcare sector, ethical principles aim to safeguard the welfare and rights of individuals. Both ethical and legal duties are owed by health service providers to prevent misuse of medical data. Collaboration between medical practitioners and data miners for data mining and matching raises ethical concerns, particularly regarding the privacy and confidentiality of individuals' sensitive information. Privacy is defined as the right of individuals to control information about themselves, protecting their integrity, reputation, and autonomy. This control extends to medical data, allowing individuals to determine who accesses their information and for what purposes. Consent is viewed as an expression of autonomy, requiring individuals to have the capacity to understand, be adequately informed, and provide voluntary consent. Autonomy also entails the right to make decisions about one's body and medical treatment. Confidentiality is crucial for protecting personal relationships and information, especially in the healthcare context. Respecting confidentiality is seen as essential for fostering trust, preventing harm, and upholding individual autonomy. Legal duties of confidentiality may arise in equity, common law, and under contract. Additionally, professional codes of conduct may impose confidentiality obligations on health service providers.

The key points regarding the ethical considerations and guidelines for research involving human participants. are as follows.

10.4.1 General Ethical Principles

Researchers and teams must protect the dignity, rights, safety, and well-being of participants. They should have the necessary qualifications, competence, and awareness of ethical, legal, and social requirements.

10.4.2 Benefit-Risk Assessment

Research should aim to maximize benefits and minimize risks to participants. Ethical Committees (ECs) are responsible for assessing and approving research plans, ensuring a favorable balance of benefits and risks.

10.4.3 Informed Consent Process

Informed consent protects individuals' autonomy to choose participation. The process involves providing relevant information, ensuring comprehension, and assuring voluntariness. The informed consent document should be reviewed and approved by the EC.

10.4.4 Categories of Risk

Research risks are categorized as less than minimal, minimal, minor increase over minimal, and more than minimal.

10.4.5 Privacy and Confidentiality

Researchers must safeguard the confidentiality of participant data.

Limitations to strict confidentiality should be explained to participants.

10.4.6 Distributive Justice

Efforts should ensure equitable distribution of benefits and burdens in research.

Vulnerable individuals/groups should not be included solely for the benefit of others.

10.4.7 Payment for Participation

Participants may be reimbursed for expenses and inconveniences, with EC approval.

10.4.8 Compensation for Research-Related Harm

Participants suffering harm are entitled to compensation, and researchers must report serious adverse events (SAEs) to the EC.

10.4.9 Ancillary Care

Participants may receive free medical care for non-research-related conditions during the study.

10.4.10 Conflict of Interest

Researchers, EC members, institutions, or sponsors must disclose and manage conflicts of interest.

10.4.11 Selection of Vulnerable and Special Groups

Vulnerable participants should be included only when directly addressing their health needs, with additional safeguards.

10.4.12 Community Engagement

Communities should be engaged throughout the research process, and community advisory boards can facilitate communication.

10.4.13 Post-Research Access and Benefit Sharing

Efforts should be made to share research findings with individuals and communities, and plans for post-research access and benefit sharing should be outlined.

10.5 Regulations and Guidelines

Data mining in reproductive health generally aligns with established principles and legal frameworks governing health care data. Some of the key considerations during the ethical data mining process are as follows.

10.5.1 Informed Consent and Data Anonymization and De-Identification

As discussed in the methodology for ethical data mining, there should be informed consent from an individual while taking and using their data for study and robust anonymization techniques should be implemented to protect individuals' identities in reproductive health datasets.

10.5.2 HIPAA Compliance (United States)

The techniques of data mining must adhere to the Health Insurance Portability and Accountability Act (HIPAA) regulations for the protection and privacy of health information and ensure that any reproductive health data collected or processed complies with HIPAA standards.

10.5.2.1 International Guidelines (e.g., WHO)

The international guidelines provided by organizations like the World Health Organization (WHO) for ethical research practices in healthcare, including reproductive health should be followed during the data collection and data mining process.

10.5.3 Ethical Review Boards and Institutional Review Boards (IRBs)

Obtain approval from relevant ethical review boards or institutional review boards overseeing research involving human subjects.

10.5.4 Security Measures

Implement stringent data security measures, including encryption and secure storage, to safeguard reproductive health data from unauthorized access.

10.5.5 Data Governance Framework

Establish a comprehensive data governance framework specific to reproductive health, outlining ethical principles, responsibilities, and processes for data management.

10.5.6 Transparency in Communication

Clearly articulate data mining practices, methodologies, and findings in public communication, ensuring transparency and avoiding misrepresentation.

10.6 Case Study: Using Data Mining Techniques to Predict Reproductive Outcomes After Varicocele Embolization

10.6.1 Introduction

Varicocele is a condition in which veins within the scrotum become enlarged in one or both testis (Arif et al. 2018). In this condition, the inflammatory pathways are triggered which is suggested to have a negative effect on spermatogenesis therefore leading to a change in sperm quality. According to the McGraw-Hill Concise Dictionary of Modern Medicine, it has been found that 40% of males who have this condition are treated for infertility.

Various treatments have been developed for varicocele among which the least invasive is radiological embolization (or varicocele embolization). This involves the introduction of coils, glue, or sclerosants into the circulation to deprive the vitality of the enlarged veins.

10.6.2 Problem

Varicocele has been observed in individuals, regardless of whether they experience infertility concerns. Therefore, it has been difficult to link varicocele with male infertility even though there is existing evidence (Su et al. 2021).

10.6.3 Objective

Due to the variability in varicocele patterns and responses to treatment, the primary objective of the study was to use data mining techniques for data analysis to predict reproductive outcomes after treatment of patients with varicocele embolization.

10.6.4 Methodology

Data Collection, Preparation, and Analysis Data analysis of 293 infertile couples was done where males had undergone varicocele embolization between January 2007 and April 2016 in Portuguese Public Hospital, the Reproductive Medicine Unit of the Centro Hospitalar e Universitário de Coimbra (CHUC). Patients who had not performed sperm analysis before varicocele embolization and the patients who did not have a partner were excluded.

A semen sample was collected after 3–5 days of sexual abstinence. It was routinely analyzed before varicocele embolization and for 3, 6, and 12 months after varicocele embolization. The sample analysis was performed by technicians according to WHO guidelines under the parameters of volume, pH, presence of leukocytes, sperm agglutination, concentration, motility, and morphology of sperm. Sperm chromatin status was also evaluated by Diff-Quik stain set to analyze the percentage of sperm with damaged DNA (Dade Behring Inc.).

Following the WHO guidelines the patients were inquired for medical records and complications were evaluated and graded according to the Clavien-Dindo classification (Dindo et al. 2004).

Primary Data Analysis The data was analyzed statistically and was viewed as primary data. The central tendencies, minimum value (Min), the value of first quartile (Q1), the value of third quartile (Q3), maximum value (Max), and standard deviation (S.D.) of each patient feature were analyzed (J. Han et al.). The chi-square, ANOVA, Kruskal-Wallis, and Mann-Whitney tests were used to assess sperm parameter values.

Data Mining Data mining involves discovering patterns within data. In this context, it's applied to analyze embolized varicocele patients and assess how their clinical features may improve based on pregnancy outcomes. The data mining techniques used were: decision tree algorithm for classification, k-means algorithm for clustering, and FP-growth algorithm for association (Tekieh and Raahemi 2015; Ahmad et al. 2015; Tomar and Agarwal 2013; Pereira et al. 2018). The CRISP-DM methodology for data mining has been depicted in Fig. 10.2.

The study utilized the Cross-Industry Standard Process for Data Mining (CRISP-DM) methodology (Chapman et al. 2000) for the mining of the data.

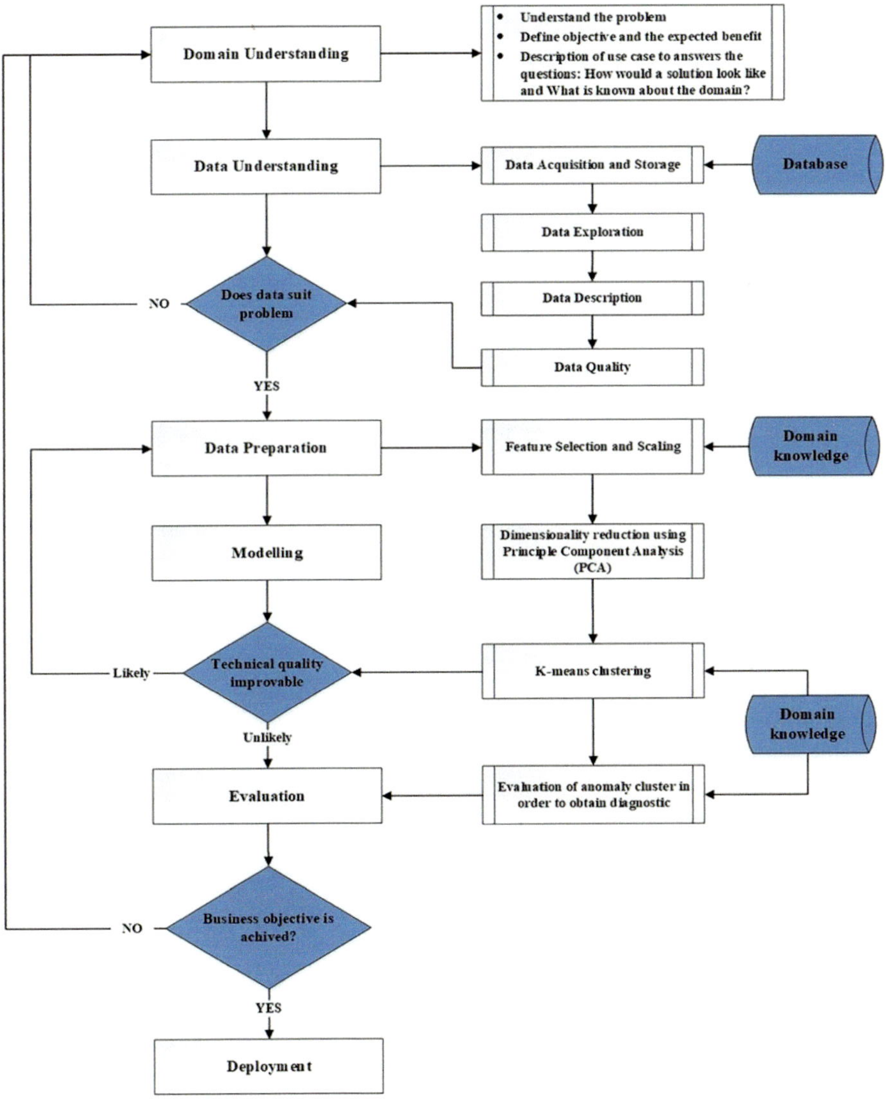

Fig. 10.2 The flow diagram depicts the CRISP-DM methodology for data mining. (Adapted from Chapman et al.) (Bekar et al. 2020)

10.7 Results

The study assessed the impact of varicocele embolization on male infertility, involving semen analysis and pregnancy outcomes. Before embolization, patients had sperm parameters below WHO reference values, with an improvement observed after embolization. Almost 80% of pregnancies occurred within a year post-embolization. Patient features significantly related to pregnancy outcome included male partner age, varicocele severity grade, and sperm parameters. Varicocele embolization success prediction was 70.59%, with specific patient characteristics influencing positive pregnancy outcomes. K-means algorithm identified data patterns showing that patients with mild to medium varicocele severity grade and normal sperm parameters were more likely to conceive. Additionally, most embolized patients did not work in hazardous occupations and had normal sperm parameters after treatment. No influence was observed from lifestyle habits or previous medical history. Furthermore, most patients reported no complications post-embolization and would undergo the procedure again.

10.8 Discussion

This study highlights the role of varicocele in male infertility and the potential benefits of varicocele embolization in improving sperm parameters and DNA integrity (Roque and Esteves 2018). The study found that varicocele embolization led to improvements in sperm concentration and DNA damage, which were associated with increased pregnancy rates (Birowo et al. 2020). The research also suggested that factors such as the age of the female partner, varicocele grade, and occupational hazards may influence reproductive outcomes. However, the study acknowledges limitations including the relatively small sample size and the lack of a control group. The authors advocate for the need for larger prospective studies to validate their findings. Despite the limitations, the study provides valuable insights into the potential benefits of varicocele correction in improving male fertility and achieving successful pregnancies.

10.9 Conclusion

The study explores the potential of using statistical and data mining techniques to identify patterns related to varicocele and its treatment success. It highlights the lack of previous research utilizing data mining to analyze varicocele databases and emphasizes its significance. The study applied k-means and FP-growth algorithms to uncover data patterns, revealing that varicocele embolization success is influenced by specific factors such as sperm motility, sperm concentration, varicocele severity, patient age, and occupation. The findings suggest that addressing male factor infertility through varicocele treatment could enhance the chances of natural conception or assisted reproductive techniques (ART). The research underscores the importance of considering minimally invasive and patient-friendly approaches for male infertility treatment, particularly in enhancing the likelihood of successful conception.

10.10 The Importance of the Ethical Board of University/College in the Process of Good Manuscript Communication

An Ethical Review Board is crucial for maintaining ethical standards in research and manuscript communication. It ensures the protection of human subjects, compliance with regulations, research integrity, confidentiality, responsible authorship, and public trust. The board reviews and approves methodologies, addresses ethical considerations in manuscripts, and ensures adherence to ethical norms throughout the research process.

An Ethical Review Board, such as an Institutional Review Board (IRB) or Ethics Committee, plays a pivotal role in ensuring the ethical conduct of research and the effective communication of its findings through manuscripts. Firstly, the board safeguards the rights, safety, and well-being of human subjects involved in the research, meticulously scrutinizing the informed consent process to ensure voluntary participation and minimize potential harm. Additionally, the board is instrumental in guiding researchers to comply with local, national, and international regulations and guidelines governing research ethics. This compliance is not only a requisite for maintaining the integrity of the institution but also contributes to the credibility of the researchers.

Moreover, the Ethical Review Board serves as a bulwark against research misconduct, including fabrication, falsification, and plagiarism, thus upholding the overall integrity of the research and the academic institution. The board's involvement extends to the evaluation of research methodology, ensuring its robustness, rigor, and scientific soundness, thereby enhancing the quality and effectiveness of manuscript communication. Confidentiality and privacy are paramount concerns addressed by the Ethical Board, particularly when handling sensitive data. This commitment fosters trust among research participants and protects their privacy. In the context of manuscript preparation, the board reviews and approves the informed consent documentation, underscoring its vital role in upholding ethical standards in research communication. Furthermore, the Ethical Board extends its oversight to the content of manuscripts, ensuring ethical considerations are adequately addressed. This includes proper acknowledgment of contributors, disclosure of conflicts of interest, and transparent reporting of results. The board also plays a crucial role in promoting responsible authorship, guiding researchers to credit those who have substantially contributed to the research, thereby fostering fairness and transparency.

Beyond the academic realm, the Ethical Review Board contributes to building and maintaining trust between the academic institution and the broader community. A reputation for ethical research enhances the credibility of the institution and its researchers, reinforcing the importance of ethical oversight in the broader societal context. Lastly, the board assists researchers in navigating legal and ethical challenges, ensuring that manuscript communication aligns with established ethical norms and regulations. In essence, the Ethical Review Board serves as a cornerstone in the research process, safeguarding ethical standards and contributing to the responsible and trustworthy communication of research findings through manuscripts (Ethical Guidelines, Institutional Regulations, Institutional Review Boards).

Acknowledgments The authors would like to acknowledge Bioinformatics Centre, Dept. of Bioscience & Biotechnology Banasthali Vidyapith to provide the computational facilities and access to the research articles. Also acknowledge the use of AI-based tools such as Quillbot and Grammarly to improve readability and summarize some parts of the text. The authors have further reviewed the text and take full responsibility for the text.

References

(2023) Digital Personal Data Protection Act 2023. https://www.meity.gov.in/writereaddata/files/Digital%20Personal%20Data%20Protection%20Act%202023.pdf

Ahmad P, Qamar S, Qasim Afser Rizvi S (2015) Techniques of data mining in healthcare: a review. IJCA 120:38–50. https://doi.org/10.5120/21307-4126

Aktar B, Rajendra KL, Clark E et al (2022) Feasibility of establishing a core set of sexual, reproductive, maternal, newborn, child, and adolescent health indicators in humanitarian settings: results from a multi-methods assessment in Bangladesh. Reprod Health 19:121. https://doi.org/10.1186/s12978-022-01424-8

Arif C, Kotoulas K, Georgellis C et al (2018) Two case reports of varicocele rupture during sexual intercourse and review of the literature. Case Rep Urol 2018:1–6. https://doi.org/10.1155/2018/4068174

Baik SM, Kim KT, Lee H, Lee JH (2023) Machine learning algorithm for early-stage prediction of severe morbidity in COVID-19 pneumonia patients based on bio-signals. BMC Pulm Med 23:121. https://doi.org/10.1186/s12890-023-02421-8

Banerjee M, Reynolds E, Andersson HB, Nallamothu BK (2019) Tree-based analysis: a practical approach to create clinical decision-making tools. Circ: Cardiovasc Qual Outcomes 12:e004879. https://doi.org/10.1161/CIRCOUTCOMES.118.004879

Bekar ET, Nyqvist P, Skoogh A (2020) An intelligent approach for data pre-processing and analysis in predictive maintenance with an industrial case study. Adv Mech Eng 12:168781402091920. https://doi.org/10.1177/1687814020919207

Bindemann M, Burton AM (2009) The role of color in human face detection. Cogn Sci 33:1144–1156. https://doi.org/10.1111/j.1551-6709.2009.01035.x

Birowo P, Tendi W, Widyahening IS et al (2020) The benefits of varicocele repair for achieving pregnancy in male infertility: a systematic review and meta-analysis. Heliyon 6:e05439. https://doi.org/10.1016/j.heliyon.2020.e05439

Bognar G (2015) Fair Innings. Bioethics 29:251–261. https://doi.org/10.1111/bioe.12101

Chapman P, Clinton J, Kerber R et al (2000) CRISP-DM 1.0. Step-by-step data mining guide. The CRISP-DM consortium. https://docplayer.net/202628-Crisp-dm-1-0-step-by-step-data-mining-guide.html

Chen IY, Pierson E, Rose S et al (2021) Ethical machine learning in healthcare. Annu Rev Biomed Data Sci 4:123–144. https://doi.org/10.1146/annurev-biodatasci-092820-114757

Chua M, Kim D, Choi J et al (2022) Tackling prediction uncertainty in machine learning for healthcare. Nat Biomed Eng 7:711–718. https://doi.org/10.1038/s41551-022-00988-x

Cossio-Gil Y, Omara M, Watson C et al (2022) The roadmap for implementing value-based healthcare in European university hospitals—consensus report and recommendations. Value Health 25:1148–1156. https://doi.org/10.1016/j.jval.2021.11.1355

Davies B (2023) Healthcare priorities: the “young” and the “old.”. Camb Q Healthc Ethics 32:174–185. https://doi.org/10.1017/S0963180122000299
Dawn AG, Balkrishnan R, Feldman SR (2008) Systematic selection bias: a cause of dramatic errors in the inference of treatment effectiveness. J Dermatol Treat 19:68–71. https://doi.org/10.1080/09546630701870780
Dindo D, Demartines N, Clavien P-A (2004) Classification of surgical complications: a new proposal with evaluation in a cohort of 6336 patients and results of a survey. Ann Surg 240:205–213. https://doi.org/10.1097/01.sla.0000133083.54934.ae
Dot G, Rafflenbeul F, Arbotto M et al (2020) Accuracy and reliability of automatic three-dimensional cephalometric landmarking. Int J Oral Maxillofac Surg 49:1367–1378. https://doi.org/10.1016/j.ijom.2020.02.015
Etges APBDS, Ruschel KB, Polanczyk CA, Urman RD (2020) Advances in value-based health-care by the application of time-driven activity-based costing for inpatient management: a systematic review. Value Health 23:812–823. https://doi.org/10.1016/j.jval.2020.02.004
Feeley TW, Landman Z, Porter ME (2020) The agenda for the next generation of health care information technology. NEJM Catalyst 1:CAT.20.0132. https://doi.org/10.1056/CAT.20.0132
Leusder M, Van Elten HJ, Ahaus K et al (2023) Protocol for improving the costs and outcomes of assistive reproductive technology fertility care pathways: a study using cost measurement and process mining. BMJ Open 13:e067792. https://doi.org/10.1136/bmjopen-2022-067792
Pereira AK, Sousa AP, Santos JR, Bernardino J (2018) Open source data mining tools evaluation using OSSpal methodology. In: Proceedings of the 13th international conference on software technologies. SCITEPRESS - Science and Technology Publications, Porto, pp 706–712
Pika A, Wynn MT, Budiono S et al (2020) Privacy-preserving process mining in healthcare. IJERPH 17:1612. https://doi.org/10.3390/ijerph17051612
Porter ME, Lee TH (2013) The strategy that will fix health care—health care and treatment. Harvard Business Review. https://hbr.org/2013/10/the-strategy-that-will-fix-health-care
Prunty JE, Jenkins R, Qarooni R, Bindemann M (2023) Ingroup and outgroup differences in face detection. Br J Psychol 114:94–111. https://doi.org/10.1111/bjop.12588
Rajkomar A, Hardt M, Howell MD et al (2018) Ensuring fairness in machine learning to advance health equity. Ann Intern Med 169:866. https://doi.org/10.7326/M18-1990
Roque M, Esteves SC (2018) Effect of varicocele repair on sperm DNA fragmentation: a review. Int Urol Nephrol 50:583–603. https://doi.org/10.1007/s11255-018-1839-4
Su JS, Farber NJ, Vij SC (2021) Pathophysiology and treatment options of varicocele: an overview. Andrologia 53. https://doi.org/10.1111/and.13576
Tekieh MH, Raahemi B (2015) Importance of data Mining in Healthcare: a survey. In: Proceedings of the 2015 IEEE/ACM international conference on advances in social networks analysis and mining 2015. ACM, Paris, pp 1057–1062
Tomar D, Agarwal S (2013) A survey on data mining approaches for healthcare. IJBSBT 5:241–266. https://doi.org/10.14257/ijbsbt.2013.5.5.25

Reproductive Health Data Mining: Case Studies

11

Sudeepti Kulshrestha, Payal Gupta, Aryan Chikara, Kashika Kapoor, Muskan Syed, Priyanka Narad, and Abhishek Sengupta

Abstract

This chapter focuses on case studies that demonstrate how approaches to data mining are used in the field of reproductive health practice and research. The focus of the chapter begins with an introduction to data mining tools and techniques which covers various aspects of several easy-to-use, free programs, such as WEKA (Waikato Environment for Knowledge Analysis), Rapid Miner, Knime, and Orange. This section discusses the pros and cons of each of these programs and their applications in the field. Further, the chapter discusses data mining pipelines and provides a general workflow for performing data mining on healthcare data. It further discusses the data mining algorithms commonly used in reproductive health research such as decision tree, random forest and support vector machines providing an example of these in research. In the final section of the chapter, two case studies are elaborated which provide a real-world illustration of the examples of data mining pipeline with reference to the reproductive health data.

Keywords

Data mining · Machine learning · Statistical analysis · Pattern recognition WEKA · Reproductive health data

S. Kulshrestha · P. Gupta · A. Chikara · K. Kapoor · M. Syed · P. Narad · A. Sengupta (✉)
Systems Biology and Data Analytics Research Lab, Amity Institute of Biotechnology, Amity University, Uttar Pradesh, Noida, India
e-mail: asengupta@amity.edu

A. Sengupta et al. (eds.), *Data-Driven Reproductive Health*,
https://doi.org/10.1007/978-981-97-7451-7_11

11.1 Introduction

Reproductive health, which covers a broad spectrum of problems about the reproductive system, its activities, and its processes, is an essential part of public health. It encompasses more than just the absence of illnesses or conditions; it also includes people's general well-being and their capacity to make decisions about their sexual orientation and reproductive systems. Many elements that fall under the general category of reproductive well-being are crucial in determining the results for public health. With the use of family planning services, people can take charge of their fertility and decide when and how many children to have. The goal of maternal health efforts is to lower the rates of maternal mortality by lowering the hazards related to pregnancy, childbirth, and postpartum care. In addition, initiatives to promote sexual health tackle problems like STIs and sexual dysfunction, encouraging better ways of thinking and acting around sexuality (Denno et al. 2015). Reducing mother and newborn mortality rates can benefit populations through improved reproductive wellness outcomes, which will enhance population health overall. Furthermore, providing women and teenagers in particular with reproductive health care and information empowers them to make decisions about their bodies and futures (Geller et al. 2018). Considering its importance, there are still obstacles in the way of guaranteeing that everyone has access to complete reproductive wellness services. These include financial constraints, societal and cultural impediments, insufficient accessibility to healthcare services, and constrained policies. Enhancing the availability of medical care, introducing comprehensive sexuality education, pushing for legislative changes, and advancing gender equality and human rights are some of the interventions meant to address these issues.

Data mining is the process of finding associations, patterns, and insights in massive datasets via a variety of statistical, machine learning, and database system approaches. It entails taking significant information out of enormous volumes of unprocessed data to find knowledge, correlations, and concealed trends that may be applied to predictive analysis and decision-making (Girija and Shashidhara 2013). Large-scale healthcare information repositories have made it more important than ever to have reliable tools for analyzing data that can provide insights that can be put to use. Investigators have worked hard over the years to improve the analysis of large datasets by utilizing statistical and data processing approaches. Among the many uses for these technologies, the diagnosis of health problems stands forth as a particularly promising area where data mining approaches have shown to be highly effective (Goel and Kumar 2023).

This chapter's goal is to examine case studies that demonstrate how approaches to data mining are used in the field of reproductive health practice and research. The chapter seeks to illustrate the various ways that data mining techniques are applied to address urgent problems and unearth important discoveries in the discipline of reproductive wellness by looking at real-world cases.

11.2 Data Mining Tools and Techniques

Data mining entails uncovering data patterns that traditional statistical exploratory data analysis methods may fail to reveal. While conventional statistics are typically regarded as the primary approach in this field, data mining serves as a complementary technique due to its distinct characteristics. Data mining, while based on mathematics, extends its application to include machine learning, database systems, and visualization, providing significant benefits compared to conventional statistical approaches. Notably, data mining excels in its ability to analyze diverse data types and perform inductive analysis, which is particularly valuable when researchers aim to understand the consequences of treatments where variables may complicate hypothesis formulation.

Data mining is a combination of machine learning, pattern recognition, and statistical methodologies to extract valuable insights from data, specifically focusing on patient information. It represents a distinct stage within the broader process of knowledge acquisition in databases, often referred to as knowledge discovery in databases (KDD). In the field of medical diagnosis, the classification system utilizes a model that is trained on the input information to accurately determine the patient's class. Data mining technologies enable the study of data and extract useful insights, which may be used by clinical obstetricians and gynecologists for diagnosis and treatment. Moreover, the use of medical data mining has potential advantages for patients in their pursuit of a comprehensive analysis of diverse clinical data.

Medical data is one of the numerous stored sets of datasets that are currently available on the Internet; due to its enormous number, it is important. It must be categorized using practical methods to be used more effectively. One of the most often used and successful categorization strategies is data mining; and several easy-to-use, free programs, such as WEKA, Rapid Miner, Knime, and Orange, are accessible (Mohi 2020).

11.2.1 WEKA

The Waikato Environment for Knowledge Analysis, or WEKA, is a flexible freely available program frequently used in the medical field for data mining projects. Despite not being specifically designed for the healthcare industry, its extensive feature set makes it quite useful in this field. WEKA flourishes in healthcare data preparation by providing methods to manage noise, outliers, and missing values—all essential for guaranteeing the quality of the data. Moreover, its feature selection methods help prevent overfitting, refine prediction models, and find relevant variables among big datasets.

By efficiently utilizing clinical data, healthcare providers may anticipate a range of outcomes from illness diagnosis to responses to medication through the use of WEKA's numerous algorithmic approaches to classification, which include decision trees, support vector machines, and neural networks (Kumar and Khatri 2017). By combining comparable patient cohorts, the tool's clustering approaches highlight important trends and make it easier to implement customized therapies or individualized treatment regimens. Furthermore, WEKA's association rule mining powers reveal complex correlations between medical data, improving comprehension of the course of a disease or the effectiveness of a treatment. Assessment and testing are essential to any data mining project, and WEKA provides strong tools to evaluate model performance and generalizability in real-world healthcare settings. Its versatility and efficacy for healthcare data analysis and research projects are further highlighted by its broad use in scientific and research settings and its smooth interaction with other tools and computer languages (Kumar and Khatri 2017).

The WEKA workbench set is intended to enable flexible and rapid testing of current techniques on new datasets. It offers comprehensive assistance for the whole experimental data mining process, which includes preparing the input data, statistically assessing learning schemes, and displaying both the learning outcome and the input data. It comes with a large selection of preprocessing tools in addition to a broad range of learning methods. Through a single interface, users may access this extensive and varied toolbox and evaluate several approaches to determine which is best suited for the given challenge (Santos-Pereira et al. 2022).

11.2.2 RapidMiner

RapidMiner is an advanced analytical tool that operates on the Java programming language. It encompasses several functionalities such as data mining, text mining, predictive analytics, and business analytics. The aforementioned technique is now the most extensively used open-source and unique methodology, having been successfully deployed in several domains (Wu et al. 2021).

The RapidMiner solution consists of five tools/editions:

(i) **RapidMiner Studio** is a software application that utilizes a graphical user interface (GUI) to enable the establishment of a comprehensive predictive analytic workflow. It incorporates a variance component function (VCF) feature that effectively manages the fundamental activities involved in data mining, such as data integration, cleaning, transformation, exploration, modeling, and validation. **RapidMiner Server** is a server for collaborative teamwork, automating tasks, deploying and integrating with other systems, and developing web-based applications.

(ii) **RapidMiner Radoop** is a collection of features for carrying out data mining in Hadoop that can speed up large-scale data analysis and help non-technical users get past the intricate nature of Spark Hadoop.

(iii) **RapidMiner Cloud** enables data mining tasks to be conducted on the cloud.

(iv) **RapidMiner Extensions** are extra features contributed by the community and include Web Mining, Text Processing, Text Analysis by AYLIEN, WEKA Extension, and Series Extension (Wu et al. 2021).

This application can interact with over 40 kinds of files, such as SAS, ARFF, and Stata, via URL; it additionally supports text documents, web pages, PDFs, HTML, and XML; it can also use MongoDB and Cassandra, two NoSQL databases; it can simulate with a broader range of modeling features and algorithms, such as decision trees, similarity calculation, clustering, market basket analysis, regression, neural networks, support vector machines, memory-based reasoning, model ensembles, and several approaches to validation and performance criteria; and it can evaluate enormous quantities of data using a variety of other implements, including Hadoop, Spark, Hive, MapReduce, Pig, and Mahout (Wu et al. 2021).

11.2.3 Orange

Orange is a Python-based open-source tool for data mining and intelligence that incorporates a graphical user interface to perform exploratory data analysis and visualization. Orange is visual programming for data mining, computer-based intelligence, and data inspection that is divided into sections. These numerous sections are often known as contraptions, including a spectrum that spans from fundamental subset decision-making and initial processing to perceptive illustration and observational assessment of learning algorithms (Mohi 2020).

It provides a visual programming interface that may be used in many different domains, such as data mining and healthcare. Orange includes capabilities that may be used for healthcare datasets for tasks including feature selection, analysis of clusters, modeling of predictions, and data imagining, even though it isn't primarily designed for the healthcare industry. Orange may be used in the healthcare industry to create prediction models for outcomes such as responses to treatment or patient readmission, identify subsets of patients according to medical or demographic characteristics, choose pertinent variables to expedite analysis, and display data to see patterns and trends. Moreover, unstructured healthcare data, such as clinical notes or medical literature, may be analyzed using Orange's text-mining capabilities to extract important information for study or clinical decision-making. Despite not being created with the healthcare industry in mind, Orange's adaptability and extensive toolkit make it a useful tool for data mining projects in a variety of industries, including the medical field (Peker et al. 2018).

In addition, Orange is capable of integrating with other graphical devices that make use of methods derived from the Focus Library and Orange modules, integrating various devices into an application via the use of visual programming techniques (Mohi 2020).

11.2.4 KNIME

Konstanz Information Miner, or KNIME, is a widely used freely available tool for data analytics, reporting, and integration in a variety of industries, especially the healthcare sector. KNIME is well known for its intuitive graphical user interface, which allows users to construct data processes visually that include pretreatment, analysis, modeling, and visualization. KNIME is a flexible tool that has several uses in data mining and analytics in the healthcare industry. Predictive modeling is one of KNIME's main uses in the medical field. Healthcare companies may create prediction models for significant results including patient readmission, illness diagnosis, and therapy response by utilizing a wide range of machine learning methods. These models provide physicians with insightful information that supports well-informed decision-making and the streamlining of patient care (Mazanetz et al. 2012). Additionally, KNIME is very good at data integration, which is important in the healthcare industry because data is frequently scattered across many sources and formats. The features of KNIME facilitate the smooth integration and preparation of various healthcare datasets, setting the stage for in-depth examination and understanding. Clinical decision assistance is an additional domain in which KNIME excels. KNIME workflows may provide real-time suggestions to healthcare practitioners by combining clinical guidelines, patient data, and predictive models. This can enhance the diagnostic, therapy, and care management procedures (Santos-Pereira et al. 2022).

KNIME's clustering and segmentation algorithms make it possible to identify different patient categories based on clinical, genetic, or demographic data through patient segmentation. These discoveries open new avenues for targeted therapies and customized medicine strategies aimed at certain patient populations. Additionally, KNIME's anomaly detection algorithms are an essential tool for the healthcare industry, helping to spot anomalies or strange trends in data, such as bogus claims or possible disease outbreaks. Maintaining healthcare systems' security and integrity depends on early anomaly identification.

11.3 Data Mining Pipeline

The growing acceptance of novel data mining techniques in bioinformatics data analysis has been fuelled by their expansion into a vital tool for understanding the huge and quickly developing landscape of biological data. With the help of these advanced methods, scientists can sort through enormous datasets from a variety of biological sources, such as proteomics, metabolomics, genomics, and more, to find hidden relationships, patterns, and insights that might not be immediately obvious when using more conventional analytical techniques. Data mining techniques are useful tools in the bioinformatics toolbox that help interpret and integrate complex biological data to improve our comprehension of basic biological phenomena and guide the development of new therapeutic approaches and clinical interventions. These techniques range from finding genetic variants linked to diseases to deciphering complex molecular pathways underlying biological processes. Every stage or phase that is involved in data mining is essential for deriving valuable conclusions from massive databases. According to the particular objectives of the data mining project and the methods used, these phases may differ somewhat (Zaki et al. 2007).

There are distinct stages in the data mining process as explained below:

(i) **Comprehending the issue**: This preliminary phase entails identifying the issue or goal of the data mining endeavor. It entails locating the data sources, comprehending the background of the study or business, and setting precise objectives and success standards.

(ii) **Data exploration**: During this phase, analysts look into the dataset to learn about its features, framework, and integrity. To find trends, outliers, and correlations in the data, methods including exploratory data analysis (EDA), data presentation, and statistical summary are used.

(iii) **Data preprocessing**: Cleaning, transforming, and preparing raw data for analysis are important steps in the data preparation process. This might entail choosing pertinent characteristics or attributes, scaling or normalizing variables, addressing outliers, and managing values that are missing.

(iv) **Model evaluation**: Following construction, models must be assessed to determine their effectiveness and capacity for generalization. To assess the predictive capability and dependability of the model, measures including accuracy, precision, recall, F1-score, and area under the curve (AUC) are used.

(v) **Model deployment**: After effective assessment, the selected approach is put into output or used to produce useful insights. This phase might include automating decision-making procedures, developing reports or representations for stakeholders, or integrating the model into already-existing systems.

(vi) **Monitoring and maintenance**: To guarantee that data mining models continue to operate at their best throughout time, ongoing monitoring and maintenance are necessary. This entails monitoring the model's effectiveness, retraining models as needed to adjust to shifting circumstances or trends in the data, and improving models with fresh data.

Additionally, the steps followed for performing data mining analysis on healthcare data have been depicted in Fig. 11.1.

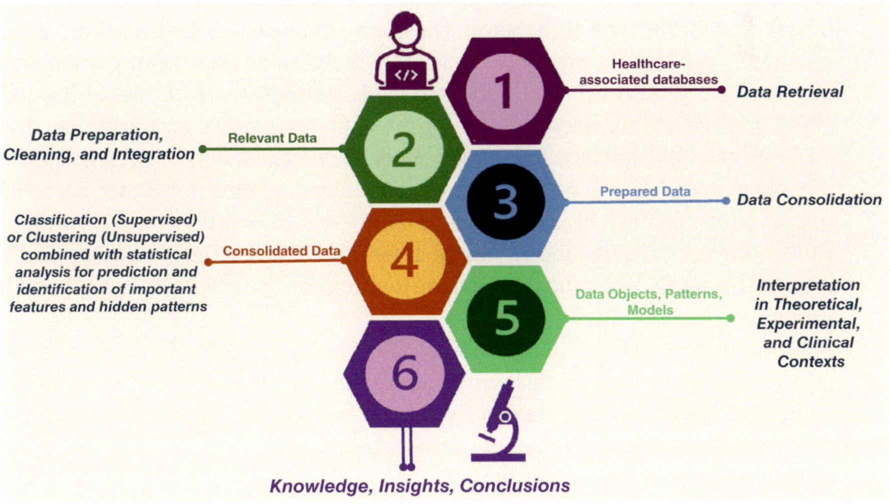

Fig. 11.1 General workflow for performing data mining on healthcare data. (Utilizing Data Mining Techniques for the Prediction of Reproductive Outcomes subsequent to Varicocele Embolization (From Sousa et al. (2021), licensed under CC-BY 4.0)

11.4 Data Mining Algorithms

Reliable clinical decision-making and risk assessment depend on the beneficial insights that data mining centered around clinical big data may generate. These objectives can be achieved with the use of data-mining methodologies (Joseph et al. 2016). Data mining utilizes two sorts of models: descriptive and predictive. Descriptive models are often used to elucidate patterns that account for data that can be easily comprehended by individuals, whilst predictive models are utilized to anticipate uncertain or possible consequences of other factors of significance. In general, a task involves the application of a model, and the description aims to predict the patterns of potential links identified in the data. As an outcome, using a descriptive model often yields a small number of groups with identical or comparable properties. Prediction is the process of estimating the value of an attribute by considering the values of other attributes, by utilizing techniques such as regression and classification (Jothi et al. 2015).

Some of the most commonly used algorithms in the data mining process are:

(i) **Decision tree:** A basic approach for classification and regression, the decision tree is structured like a flowchart, with the root node at the top and each node representing a test on an attribute, branches representing attribute outputs, and leaf nodes representing classes or class distributions. The decision tree model, which is categorized as a regression tree for regression problems and a classification tree for classification tasks, has demonstrated its efficacy in clinical applications. For example, it demonstrated better prediction power using real clinical data, outperforming traditional logistic regression models in prognostic assessments of breast cancer patients. Furthermore, the decision tree has shown useful in several therapeutic settings, including the diagnosis of kidney stones, the prediction of the risk of sudden cardiac arrest, and the identification of risk factors for type II diabetes. These investigations make use of the decision tree's capacity to investigate variable interactions and group participants into uniform groups according to observable attributes, which makes it especially appropriate for decision algorithms with comparable architectures. The decision tree has advantages, however the fact that it builds trees based on recursive observation separation shows that managing data imbalance has to be improved to increase model precision. However, compared to standard algorithms, the decision tree model has clear benefits and practical utility for building clinical prediction models and investigating disease risk factors and patient prognosis (Li et al. 2019).

(ii) **Random forest (RF):** Employing a set of decision trees, the RF method is one prominent example of an ensemble learning application. Using the bootstrap technique, decision trees created by randomly selecting sample sets from the training set result in a diverse set of trees. Next, predictions are obtained using a majority vote or ensemble average. One of RF's main benefits is that it randomly selects predictor variables at every decision tree node, which effectively lowers correlation across the trees and raises the accuracy of ensemble predictions. By addressing the overfitting problem that single decision tree models face, prediction accuracy is subsequently increased. The ability of RF to reliably distinguish between in-hospital mortality among sepsis patients admitted to the emergency room—a crucial area needing exact forecasting techniques in a hectic and fast-paced setting. Their results proved the superiority of RF over standard emergency care techniques, allowing a wider variety of clinical factors to be evaluated and revealing predictors that would have been missed with traditional modeling approaches. Furthermore, innovative methodologies such as random survival forests provide promising avenues for survival analysis, particularly in the field of clinical cancer, enabling the development of personalized treatment strategies that will be advantageous for patients (Wongvibulsin et al. 2020).

(iii) **Support vector machine (SVM):** SVM is an innovative approach for classification and prediction, developed by Cortes and Vapnik. It provides a data-driven method without making any presumptions about the pattern of distribution of the data. Finding a separation boundary, often referred to as a hyperplane, is the main goal of SVM in case classification. This is especially helpful when dealing with high-dimensional data or datasets that have small sample sizes. SVM was used to build a predictive model in research that dealt with medication compliance in patients with heart failure. This allowed for the successful avoidance of the problem of a large number of input variables about the observations that were available. Furthermore, SVMs are excellent at handling the complexities involved in chronic and complicated illnesses, where many risk variables, such as gene-gene and gene-environment interactions, need to be taken into account yet processes are still unclear. Due to their robust ability to differentiate, SVMs have the potential to be used as a classification technique for identifying individuals with such diseases. Nevertheless, a notable drawback of SVMs is their tendency to require a substantial amount of effort and resources, often resulting in inefficiencies when dealing with large observation sets. Notwithstanding this drawback, the application of SVMs in clinical research highlights their potential to improve predictive modeling and deepen our understanding of the dynamics of complicated diseases (Gaye et al. 2021).

(iv) **Competitive risk model:** Survival analysis in clinical research relies on the core methods of the Cox proportional hazards model and Kaplan-Meier marginal regression. Survival analysis has traditionally concentrated on one outcome, usually the patient's survival time. Several endpoints, however, frequently coexist in clinical research, creating a rivalry between these endpoints and producing competitive risk data. Because there are competing concerns, relying solely on one endpoint analysis approach in these situations may result in skewed estimates of endpoint event probability. For right-censored survival data with many endpoints, the competitive risk model provides reliable estimates of cumulative incidence, based on conventional statistical theories about data distribution (Klein 2010).

11.5 Case Study 1: Utilizing Data Mining Techniques for the Prediction of Reproductive Outcomes Subsequent to Varicocele Embolization (Sousa et al. 2021)

11.5.1 Overview

A retrospective analysis was performed on a dataset comprising 293 couples experiencing infertility, defined as partners who were unable to conceive after 1 year of recurring sexual activity. These couples had male spouses who underwent varicocele embolization in Portugal between January 2007 and April 2016, to enhance the likelihood of pregnancy for the couples. The research excluded patients who did not have a spouse and those who had not had sperm analysis before the varicocele embolization.

This study included evaluating how well specific clinical aspects had improved, forecasting treatment success based on pregnancy results, and spotting data trends that would help with future varicocele research and better post-therapy patient care. The researchers used a variety of statistical tools, including classical approaches, together with widely used data mining techniques in the healthcare industry to achieve these goals.

11.5.2 Data Mining

The research used prevalent data mining methods in the healthcare field, such as decision tree classification, k-means clustering, and FP-growth association since these approaches are seldom used in medical and healthcare domains.

The six steps of the cross-industry standard procedure for data mining project (CRISP-DM) methodology, which allows for iterative execution, were adhered to during the data mining process. Understanding business objectives and data mining goals, gathering and analyzing data while confirming its quality, preparing data by sorting, cleaning, and formatting it, selecting suitable data mining techniques, creating models, and assessing it using performance metrics are all included in these phases. Ultimately, outcomes are disclosed to stakeholders throughout the deployment phase.

The modeling phase included well-recognized methods for data mining in the healthcare domain, including association, clustering, and classification. Hence, the RapidMiner data mining platform was used to apply the decision tree technique for classification, the k-means algorithm for clustering, and the FP-growth algorithm for association.

11.5.3 Results

According to semen data mining analysis, the sperm concentration and progressive motility of the patients were found to be below the standard standards set by the World Health Organization (WHO) before embolization. Moreover, sperm exhibited chromatin fragmentation, suggesting compromised chromatin integrity in sperm. The sperm parameters showed significant improvement after embolization 3 months post-treatment. The only parameter that did not exhibit significant improvement after 1 year was sperm concentration. Following embolization, there was an observed increase in chromatin integrity, but it remained higher than the commonly accepted reference value of 32%.

11.5.4 Discussion

Following therapy, around 47% of those receiving treatment became pregnant, either naturally or with the use of ART, and 80% of them did so within the first year following embolization. In a similar vein, several reports have indicated that varicocele repair led to higher rates of pregnancy and live births. The researchers' work revealed that reproductive results are related to both the characteristics of the sperm identified before treatment and the improvements gained after embolization. In addition, additional factors that may be significant include the female spouse's age, the grade of varicocele, and the possibility of a hazardous career as indicated by the decision tree and/or cluster analysis. Their prospective predictive values had never been evaluated, even though several research has examined the relationship between varicocele/varicocele therapy and several pertinent characteristics, including sperm parameters.

By using several algorithms, such as k-means and FP-growth, the researchers were able to find interesting patterns in the data. These results imply that there is a favorable correlation between several parameters and the success of varicocele embolization, as determined by obtaining pregnancy and live delivery. The sperm progressive motility was normal before treatment; the sperm concentration was normal following medical care; the varicocele severity grade was moderate to low; the male patient was younger; and the male patient's occupation did not involve working with possibly toxic substances or environments.

Taking into account these findings and the fact that intracytoplasmic sperm injection (ICSI) is still a treatment option for cases of severe infertility affecting men, it is crucial to look at the male factors to increase the likelihood of conception, either naturally or with the use of ART. This is especially important when there is a simple, non-invasive, and patient-friendly way to give the medication.

11.6 Case Study 2: Employing Data Mining Techniques to Predict the Implantation Outcome of In Vitro Fertilization and Intracytoplasmic Sperm Injection (Hafiz et al. 2017)

11.6.1 Overview

When it comes to clinical and demographic traits, IVF and ICSI share a lot of similarities. According to a recent study carried out in Iran, the average population affected by infertility is 10.9%. Of the patients who visited different infertility clinics around the nation, 78.4% had primary infertility and 21.6% had secondary infertility. According to the study, 44.5% of instances were linked to female factors, 17.1% to a combination of both, and 8.1% of cases were still unaccounted for. Of the cases, 34.0% were linked to male causes. Notably, among the female reasons examined in this study, ovulatory dysfunction turned out to be the most common etiological component.

In this study, five established data mining classification methods were used utilizing the dataset. The training and testing processes were carried out using fivefold cross-validation. The primary objective of this research was to ascertain the most effective prediction model for forecasting the likelihood of success in IVF/ICSI procedures for each couple by evaluating many classifiers. Moreover, the crucial factors that most accurately predict the effectiveness of assisted reproductive technology (ART) for couples experiencing infertility were found.

The census technique was used to collect 486 patient records and 29 variables from the IVF/ICSI dataset. Each person is assigned a unique identity that reflects their positive or negative status. Computed for the classifiers were mean accuracy, receiver operating characteristic (ROC) curve, sensitivity, specificity, as well as positive and negative predictive values. The analysis included advanced classifiers such as RF, adaptive boosting, recursive partitioning (RPART), and one-nearest neighbor.

11.6.2 Data Mining

A collection of 486 annotated records with 29 variables was assembled from Shiraz, Iran, between 2009 and 2015. There were 355 negative implantations and 131 positive implantations in this dataset; the higher number of negative samples led to a highly skewed distribution. Trained staff members retrieved the necessary variables for analysis from paper-based medical records and then added them to the dataset for computer modeling.

In this work, a strategy was used to substitute the values that were missing for numerical features with the median and replace the mode of each column for categorical characteristics, given a dataset that had skewed distributions of missing values. The research included contemporary techniques, including SVM, RPART, RF, Adaptive Boosting (AdaBoost), and 1NN, to conduct informed decision-making on

IVF/ICSI outcomes. In order to ascertain the probability of each option rule and choose the most effective alternative for prediction, a comparison was conducted among these models. The implementation of these classifiers was carried out using R version 3.2.3, and their validation followed a fivefold stratified cross-validation approach.

11.6.3 Results

According to their results, RPART and RF fared better than other classifiers in terms of NPV, PPV, and specificity. While RF performed well in categorizing negative instances, RPART performed better in predicting positive cases. In the confusion matrices of both models, there were fewer false negatives, which contributed to the higher NPV in RPART, while a smaller number of false positives was the cause of the higher PPV value in RF. Adaboost performed better than SVM and 1NN overall, especially when it came to sensitivity. SVM showed a much lower specificity value than 1NN, although having a greater specificity than 1NN. Furthermore, although RPART indicated a moderate rise, RF revealed a huge increase in the positive likelihood ratio, indicating a significant increase in the chance of pregnancy. The remaining models, however, produced little gains. All classifiers showed negative likelihood ratios between 0.5 and 1, which suggested a slight drop in the likelihood of pregnancy.

The findings of the current research demonstrate that RF and RPART exhibited superior performance compared to prior pregnancy prediction methods. The research identified the woman's age, the number of generated embryos, and the serum estradiol levels on the day of hCG injection as the three most influential criteria for the success of IVF/ICSI.

11.6.4 Discussion

The current study has a drawback in that it only focused on a subset of data mining approaches, leaving out conventional prediction models like Templeton, logistic regression, and Bayesian methods from the comparison. The main limitation of logistic regression is that it assumes dataset components to be independent of one another, which may not apply to variables that show an inverse connection, such as follicle-stimulating hormone (FSH) and anti-Müllerian hormone (AMH). In addition, the age of a woman has been shown to correlate with factors such as FSH, AMH, oocyte count, and embryo quality, which further undermines the independence assumption.

Future research should include classical predictive models in addition to the data mining models examined in this paper to guarantee a more thorough comparison. Moreover, it is essential to create techniques that can effectively address class imbalance, particularly for classifiers that are very responsive to fluctuations in class distribution. Predictive studies in this sector would be substantially improved, ideally, by the creation of a global database tracking the results of IVF, ICSI, and assisted reproductive technology (ART) across all healthcare establishments worldwide. A database of this kind would make it easier to provide results that are more similar and universal, which would lessen the variation in ART success that is seen between research sites and strengthen the basis for clinical decision-making.

11.7 Conclusion

Public health revolves around reproductive health, which includes family planning, maternal health, and promoting sexual and reproductive health. Ensuring access to comprehensive reproductive health care promotes gender equality, social advancement, and individual well-being. Reproductive health researchers are increasingly using data mining techniques to glean insightful information from huge databases. These methods are useful for doing predictive studies and finding trends, especially when it comes to things like the results of infertility treatments. Utilizing data mining techniques in reproductive health research has great potential to improve patient outcomes and healthcare delivery by deepening our understanding of intricate biology and clinical processes. Researchers may find hidden patterns, pinpoint predictive elements, and create more accurate models for infertility diagnosis, treatment optimization, and result prediction in assisted reproductive technologies (ART) by utilizing huge and diverse datasets through data mining. Moreover, data mining makes it easier to combine information from many sources, including clinical, genetic, and environmental data, allowing for a more thorough and individualized approach to reproductive health care. Data mining can spur innovation, improve clinical decision-making, and eventually increase reproductive health research and practice by drawing useful insights from massive volumes of data. Data mining has the potential to have a significant influence on reproductive health research by revolutionizing patient care, diagnosis, and therapy. Data mining can enhance prediction models for ART results, provide individualized approaches to reproductive healthcare, and reveal new insights into the underlying causes of infertility by utilizing sophisticated analytical tools like machine learning and pattern recognition. Class imbalance and data heterogeneity are two methodological issues that should be addressed in the field's future directions. Multidisciplinary approach integration and the creation of cooperative research projects should also be encouraged. Furthermore, establishing thorough databases for reproductive health outcomes and putting data-sharing procedures in place will be essential for encouraging innovation and developing evidence-based practices in the industry. All things considered, data mining's continuous development and application in the field of reproductive health show great potential for enhancing patient outcomes and influencing the direction of this crucial area of medicine in the future.

Acknowledgments The authors would like to acknowledge the use of AI-based tools such as Quillbot and Grammarly to improve readability and summarize some parts of the text. The authors have further reviewed the text and take full responsibility for the text.

References

Denno DM, Hoopes AJ, Chandra-Mouli V (2015) Effective strategies to provide adolescent sexual and reproductive health services and to increase demand and community support. J Adolesc Health 56:S22–S41. https://doi.org/10.1016/j.jadohealth.2014.09.012

Gaye B, Zhang D, Wulamu A (2021) Improvement of support vector machine algorithm in big data background. Math Probl Eng 2021:1–9. https://doi.org/10.1155/2021/5594899

Geller SE, Koch AR, Garland CE et al (2018) A global view of severe maternal morbidity: moving beyond maternal mortality. Reprod Health 15:98. https://doi.org/10.1186/s12978-018-0527-2

Girija DKS, Shashidhara MS (2013) Data mining techniques used for uterus fibroid diagnosis and prognosis. In: 2013 International mutli-conference on automation, computing, communication, control and compressed sensing (iMac4s). IEEE, Kottayam, pp 372–376

Goel H, Kumar D (2023) Data mining in healthcare using machine learning techniques. In: 2023 International conference on sustainable computing and smart systems (ICSCSS). IEEE, Coimbatore, pp 25–29

Hafiz P, Nematollahi M, Boostani R, Jahromi BN (2017) Predicting implantation outcome of in vitro fertilization and intracytoplasmic sperm injection using data mining techniques. Int J Fertil Steril 11. https://doi.org/10.22074/ijfs.2017.4882

Joseph SR, Hlomani H, Letsholo K (2016) Data mining algorithms: an overview. IJCT 15:6806–6813. https://doi.org/10.24297/ijct.v15i6.1615

Jothi N, Rashid NA, Husain W (2015) Data mining in healthcare—a review. Procedia Comput Sci 72:306–313. https://doi.org/10.1016/j.procs.2015.12.145

Klein JP (2010) Competing risks. WIREs Comp Stats 2:333–339. https://doi.org/10.1002/wics.83

Kumar N, Khatri S (2017) Implementing WEKA for medical data classification and early disease prediction. In: 2017 3rd International conference on Computational Intelligence & Communication Technology (CICT). IEEE, Ghaziabad, pp 1–6

Li H, Wu TT, Yang DL et al (2019) Decision tree model for predicting in-hospital cardiac arrest among patients admitted with acute coronary syndrome. Clin Cardiol 42:1087–1093. https://doi.org/10.1002/clc.23255

Mazanetz MP, Marmon RJ, CBT R, Morao I (2012) Drug discovery applications for KNIME: an open source data mining platform. Curr Top Med Chem 12:1965–1979. https://doi.org/10.2174/156802612804910331

Mohi ZR (2020) Orange data mining as a tool to compare classification algorithms. Dijlah J 3:13–23

Peker M, Özkaraca O, Şaşar A, (2018) Use of orange data mining toolbox for data analysis in clinical decision making: the diagnosis of diabetes disease. In: Expert system techniques in biomedical science practice. IGI Global, p 280. https://doi.org/10.2174/10.4018/978-1-5225-5149-2.ch007.

Santos-Pereira J, Gruenwald L, Bernardino J (2022) Top data mining tools for the healthcare industry. J King Saud Univ Comput Inform Sci 34:4968–4982. https://doi.org/10.1016/j.jksuci.2021.06.002

Sousa AP, Santos-Pereira J, Freire MJ et al (2021) Using data mining to assist in predicting reproductive outcomes following varicocele embolization. JCM 10:3503. https://doi.org/10.3390/jcm10163503

Wongvibulsin S, Wu KC, Zeger SL (2020) Clinical risk prediction with random forests for survival, longitudinal, and multivariate (RF-SLAM) data analysis. BMC Med Res Methodol 20:1. https://doi.org/10.1186/s12874-019-0863-0

Wu W-T, Li Y-J, Feng A-Z et al (2021) Data mining in clinical big data: the frequently used databases, steps, and methodological models. Mil Med Res 8:44. https://doi.org/10.1186/s40779-021-00338-z

Zaki MJ, Karypis G, Yang J (2007) Data Mining in Bioinformatics (BIOKDD). Algorithms Mol Biol 2:4. https://doi.org/10.1186/1748-7188-2-4

12 Future Directions and Emerging Trends in Reproductive Health

Yegna Subramanian Jambunath, Kunal D. Patil, K. S. Kishor Bharadwaj, D. B. Santosh Bhargav, and T. J. Ramnath Babu

Abstract

The revolution in Reproductive Health and Medicine is being propelled by the integration of Machine Learning (ML) and Artificial Intelligence (AI) technologies, marking a new era of personalized patient care and enhanced outcomes. At the forefront of this transformation is the development of a centralized Data Hub, which amalgamates multifaceted data sources from Assisted Reproductive Technology (ART) processes. This consolidation facilitates profound data analysis, fostering informed decision-making and insightful research. Furthermore, the advent of ML Decision Support Systems introduces precision at critical intervention junctures within the ART sequence, significantly elevating success rates. Large Language Models (LLMs) tailored for reproductive medicine enhance patient communication and streamline data handling, presenting a novel approach to patient-centric care. Federated Learning emerges as a pivotal technology, championing data privacy and collaborative research without compromising patient confidentiality. Other notable advancements include the application of Blockchain for secure data transactions and Genome Sequence Modelling, paving the way for genetic insights in reproductive health. The journey from Research to Production encapsulates the challenges of transitioning these ground-breaking technologies into practical clinical applications, emphasizing the need for strategic implementation to fully harness their potential in reproductive healthcare settings. This chapter discusses these emerging trends and directions, detailing the processes and technologies that are setting the course for the future of Reproductive Health and Medicine.

Y. S. Jambunath (✉) · K. D. Patil · K. S. Kishor Bharadwaj · D. B. Santosh Bhargav · T. J. Ramnath Babu
SpOvum Technologies Private Limited, Bengaluru, India
e-mail: yegna.s@spovum.com

A. Sengupta et al. (eds.), *Data-Driven Reproductive Health*,
https://doi.org/10.1007/978-981-97-7451-7_12

Keywords

Data hub · Blockchain · ML decision support system · LLM · Federated learning Genome sequence modelling · MLOps · LLMOps

12.1 Introduction

12.1.1 Data Hub

A "Data Hub" in ART is a central platform where data originating from different sources, such as Double witnessing systems, Computer Aided Semen Analyzer (CASA), Lab parameters monitoring and alarming systems, Time Lapse Embryo Monitoring Systems (TL-EMS), Programmable Intra-cytoplasmic Sperm Injection (ICSI) manipulators, New-generation technologies that can collect additional layers of data non-invasively (like micro-gripper based techniques to gather mechanical properties of oocytes and embryos during micromanipulation) along with Human input data, is gathered, consolidated, and organized. This hub serves as a foundational component for effective data management, analysis, report generation, and research in the field of reproductive medicine, enabling comprehensive insights and informed decision-making.

12.1.2 ML Decision Support Systems

Implementing specialized models at each intervention point in the ART process for informed decision-making and improved outcomes.

12.1.3 LLM for Reproductive Medicine

Leveraging pre-trained models tailored for Reproductive Medicine and harnessing that using LLM Operations to enhance patient communication, data analysis, and information extraction.

12.1.4 Federated Learning in Reproductive Health and Medicine

Embracing data privacy and security through collaborative model training while safeguarding patient confidentiality, fostering collective advancements in ART research and patient care.

12.1.5 Other Emerging Technologies

Genome Sequence Modelling and Blockchain for Reproductive Health and Medicine.

12.1.6 Research to Production

This section delves into the journey of transitioning cutting-edge technologies from the research phase to clinical application in the field of reproductive medicine. The focus is on the challenges and considerations associated with the adoption of these technologies and the specific requirements for successful implementation in reproductive healthcare settings.

12.2 Data-Driven Approaches in Reproductive Health

Advancements in bioinformatics and machine learning offer unprecedented opportunities to revolutionize reproductive health through data-driven approaches. The collection and organization of data about reproductive health stand as a cornerstone for shaping the future well-being of citizens, offering personalized treatments, establishing robust health protocols, and integrating evolving technologies. This pivotal requirement hinges on the acquisition of relevant data from trusted sources, employing the right data acquisition technologies, and upholding principles of transparency, anonymity, structured storage, authorized access, and data availability. The collaboration among Government bodies, Academia, Research Organizations, and Private Institutions becomes imperative to effectively gather and host such comprehensive data. Ensuring the fundamental priority of patient consent for the collection and anonymous storage of health-related data is integral to the ethical underpinning of this endeavor.

12.2.1 Comprehensive Data Collection in Reproductive Health

In the pursuit of understanding and improving reproductive health outcomes, a multitude of data types must be gathered, including but not limited to clinical records, genetic information, environmental exposures, lifestyle factors, and imaging data. For instance, studies have shown the significance of genetic profiles in understanding infertility issues, while integrating lifestyle and environmental factors is crucial in comprehending the broader context influencing reproductive health. Environmental factors within the fertility clinic setting can significantly impact the success rates and outcomes of In Vitro Fertilization (IVF) procedures. These factors encompass various aspects of the clinic environment, protocols, and practices that can influence the quality of care and the success of fertility treatments. The links to datasets numbered (Rana 2024; FP 2030 2024; NIMH Data Archive 2024) represent sources of comprehensive data collection. Each link provides access to a distinct dataset, showcasing the variety and depth of information available for further analysis. These datasets could support to building of useful applications like a dashboard tool (Davis 2024) for the public where users can explore oocyte and sperm donor information since 1991.

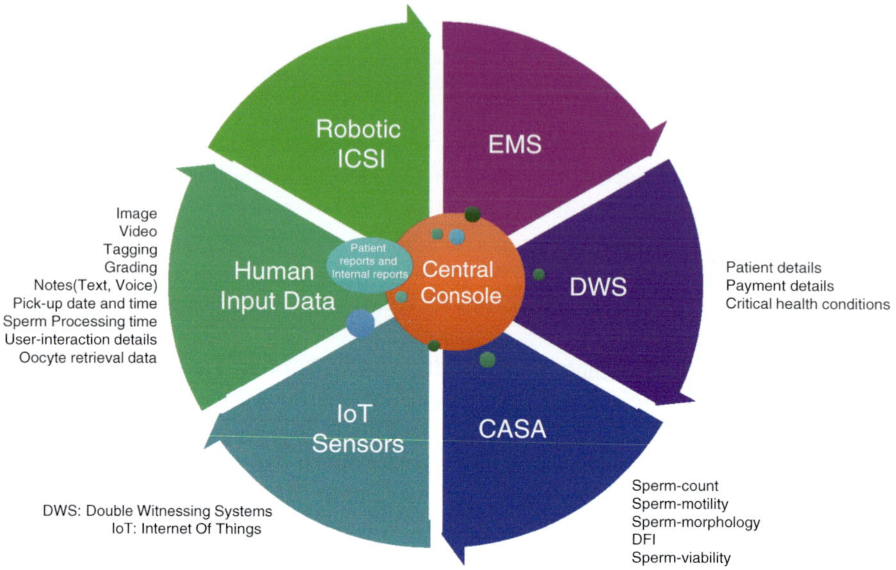

Fig. 12.1 "Data Hub" classification in ART, which serves as a critical platform aggregating and structuring data from a wide array of sources

12.2.2 Data Hub

The idea of Data Collection and Integration leads to the "Data Hub" (Fig. 12.1) in ART, which serves as a critical platform, aggregating and structuring data from a wide array of sources. By collating this diverse range of information, the hub plays an essential role in the effective management of data, facilitating the generation of detailed reports, thorough analysis, and supporting research in reproductive medicine. This comprehensive approach to data integration is pivotal for deriving meaningful insights and aiding in informed decision-making in the field. The Data Hub can be effectively achieved through a dual-method approach, encompassing both Local and Central Data Collection. Each method plays a distinct yet complementary role in the overall data management and analysis process.

12.2.2.1 Local Data Collection

At the local level, individual clinics and laboratories serve as primary data collection points. These entities are typically private and operate with their own set of protocols and equipment. Here, ML models are developed and deployed to meet specific laboratory requirements. These models are tailored to address unique challenges and objectives, such as optimizing embryo selection or improving success rates of specific ART procedures.

The local data hubs focus on the following:

- **Gathering Lab-Specific Data:** This includes patient data, procedure outcomes, equipment performance, and environmental conditions within the lab.
- **Developing Custom ML Models:** These models are designed to interpret and utilize local data effectively, providing insights and predictive analytics specific to the clinic's operations.
- **Ensuring Data Privacy:** Local hubs handle sensitive patient data, necessitating stringent privacy and security measures.

12.2.2.2 Central Data Hub

The Central Data Hub operates on a broader scale, encompassing data from multiple local hubs. It is a collaborative effort involving government bodies, academic institutions, clinics, and private entities. The central hub's objectives include the following:

- **Standardizing Data Management and Sharing:** It establishes uniform protocols for data sharing and management, akin to the NIH's genomic data sharing policy, ensuring consistency and compatibility across different entities.
- **Facilitating Data Exchange:** The hub enables the sharing of anonymized data, allowing for broader research and analysis while maintaining individual privacy.
- **Deploying and Refining ML Models:** Centralized data allows for the development of more sophisticated and comprehensive ML models that benefit from a wider dataset, potentially leading to more generalized and robust solutions in ART.

12.2.3 Federated Learning: A Solution for Privacy and Collaboration

In the context of both local and central data repositories, federated learning emerges as a potent solution for maintaining privacy while leveraging collective data insights. Federated learning is a machine learning approach where models are trained across multiple decentralized devices (or local data repositories) holding local data samples, without exchanging them. For a more in-depth understanding of how federated learning facilitates the implementation of the central hub, the Federated Learning in Reproductive Health and Medicine section will delve into specific applications and methodologies of federated learning in the context of reproductive health and ART.

12.2.4 Infrastructure and Governance for Data Storage

Storage and maintenance of this diverse array of data require robust infrastructure and stringent protocols to ensure security and accessibility. Cloud-based solutions, secure servers, and encrypted storage mechanisms are deployed while adhering to stringent access controls and encryption methodologies. Institutions and designated entities undertaking data storage and maintenance are obligated to comply with rigorous data governance policies to safeguard sensitive patient information. The accuracy and reliability of the gathered data are contingent upon the sources utilized. Electronic Health Records (EHRs), genetic databases, wearable devices, image data, and IoT sensors constitute primary sources, demanding continuous validation and verification processes to uphold data accuracy and credibility. Collaborations with reputable institutions and constant vigilance against data drift or degradation ensure the integrity of the datasets used for analysis and modeling purposes. The paramount concern in this data-intensive landscape is ensuring patient privacy, confidentiality, and anonymity. Stringent adherence to privacy laws such as (Ministry of Law and Justice (Legislative Department) 2023) is fundamental. Implementing anonymization techniques, differential privacy methods, and data de-identification protocols serve to mitigate the risks of data breaches and preserve patient confidentiality.

12.2.5 Blockchain's Role in Reproductive Health Data Management

Towards addressing this, blockchain technology, renowned for its decentralized, transparent, and secure nature, holds immense promise in revolutionizing the management of sensitive reproductive health data. When coupled with ML, it presents a formidable combination that enhances the potential of data-driven approaches within the realm of reproductive health.

Blockchain technology was outlined in the groundbreaking white paper "Bitcoin: A Peer-to-Peer Electronic Cash System," by an enigmatic figure known as Satoshi Nakamoto marks a pivotal milestone in the realm of digital or cryptocurrencies, notably Bitcoin (Nakamoto 2008). Beyond Bitcoin, blockchain found expansion in Ethereum, as detailed in Vitalik Buterin's white paper (Buterin 2015). Ethereum introduced smart contracts, self-executing contracts with the terms directly written into code, revolutionizing the possibilities for Decentralized Applications (DApps). In the acclaimed work authored by Don Tapscott and Alex Tapscott (Tapscott and Tapscott 2016) the transformative impact of blockchain is vividly explored, highlighting its pivotal role in reshaping traditional business frameworks, and enabling decentralized transactions in the fields of supply chain management and healthcare to governance.

12.2.6 Enhancing Patient Privacy and Data Integrity Through Blockchain

In the context of reproductive health, where preserving the confidentiality of patient information is paramount, the decentralized architecture of blockchain ensures heightened security (Iansiti and Lakhani 2017; Kuo et al. 2017; Mettler 2016). Its immutable ledger system guarantees data integrity, making records resistant to tampering or unauthorized alterations. This not only safeguards patient information but also fosters trust among healthcare providers and patients alike by providing a transparent and auditable trail of data modifications (Gordon and Catalini 2018). The collaboration of blockchain and ML can enable patient-centric control and ethical handling of sensitive health information. Blockchain's smart contracts empower patients to dictate specific conditions under which their data can be accessed or used, ensuring explicit and transparent consent mechanisms. Meanwhile, ML algorithms can leverage this data to provide tailored insights and recommendations, supporting clinicians in making informed decisions and optimizing treatment strategies.

12.2.7 Data Relevance and Standardization in Reproductive Health

Determining the relevance of data is a collaborative endeavor involving medical professionals, researchers, and data scientists. This necessitates meticulous decision-making to discern which data elements are pivotal for predictive models, pattern recognition, and tailored interventions. Standardizing data formats using established healthcare data standards like HL7 or FHIR (Fast Healthcare Interoperability Resources) ensures seamless interoperability and facilitates the integration of disparate datasets (Gliklich et al. 2020). Employing standardized vocabularies and ontologies aids in organizing and structuring data, enabling comprehensive analyses and informed decision-making processes.

12.2.8 Conclusion

The Data Hub in ART represents much more than a mere repository of information. It is a dynamic and integral tool that significantly enhances the quality and effectiveness of reproductive healthcare. Local and Central Data Repositories in ART represent two tiers of data management and utilization, each playing a distinct yet interconnected role. The effective use of these repositories is crucial for advancing reproductive medicine while ensuring privacy and confidentiality, a challenge that can be effectively addressed through federated learning approaches.

The collection of high-quality data through both local and central collection methods, can contribute to the development of sophisticated ML models, which in turn can lead to the creation of advanced decision support systems. The ML-driven decision support systems are elaborated in the next section.

12.3 ML Decision Support System

12.3.1 Why ML Decision Support System?

12.3.1.1 Human-Machine Teaming in ART

The synergy between human expertise and machine intelligence, often referred to as Human-Machine Teaming, offers unprecedented opportunities to enhance the efficacy and precision of ART. This collaboration can lead to improved decision-making processes, especially in complex scenarios where human intuition and machine accuracy can complement each other.

Example: An embryologist working alongside an ML-based system can more accurately determine the viability of embryos, blending their experiential knowledge with data-driven insights provided by the ML model.

12.3.1.2 Breaking the Saturation Barrier in Success Rates

The current plateau in success rates of ART procedures can be attributed to the limitations of traditional methodologies. ML, with its ability to analyze vast datasets, can uncover hidden patterns, and offers a path to break through this saturation. By integrating ML into ART, we can potentially unlock new insights and strategies that could increase success rates significantly.

12.3.2 ML Intervention: A Journey from Clinic Visit to Successful Delivery

The journey of a patient through the ART process is intricate, involving multiple departments and decision points. Machine Learning (ML) plays a pivotal role at each of these stages, ensuring personalized and optimized treatment. Let's explore this journey and the ML interventions at each decision-making juncture.

12.3.2.1 Initial Consultation and Patient Profiling

- **ML Models:**
  - Fertility Predictor
  - Lifestyle-Fertility Correlation Model
- **ML Intervention:** At the patient's first clinic visit, ML models analyze medical histories, genetic information, and lifestyle factors. Predictive analytics help in creating a comprehensive profile that guides subsequent treatment decisions.
- **How They Work:**
  - These models analyze a patient's medical history, genetic data, and lifestyle factors to identify patterns and risk factors associated with fertility issues.
  - **Example:** A Fertility Predictor model can consider a wide range of variables (age, medical history, genetic markers, lifestyle habits) and predict the likelihood of certain fertility issues or the best approach for treatment.

12.3.2.2 Diagnostic Tests and Analysis

- **ML Models:**
  - Neural Networks
  - Principal Component Analysis (PCA)
  - Cluster Analysis
- **ML Intervention:** Diagnostic data, including hormonal levels and ultrasound results, are fed into ML models. These models provide insights into potential fertility issues and suggest customized treatment pathways.
- **How They Work:**

- Neural Networks, particularly deep learning models, are adept at processing complex medical data. They can interpret hormonal levels and ultrasound imagery to identify underlying conditions affecting fertility. PCA and Cluster Analysis can be used to find correlations and groupings in the data that might not be immediately apparent, providing deeper insights for personalized treatment plans.
- **Example in Hormonal Analysis:** Consider a dataset containing various hormonal levels (like FSH, LH, estrogen, and progesterone) from numerous patients undergoing fertility treatments. PCA can reduce this complex dataset to a few principal components that capture the most significant variation in hormone levels. This simplification can help identify patterns or anomalies in hormonal profiles that could be indicative of specific fertility issues.
- **Example in Ultrasound Imagery:** Ultrasound images of ovaries and follicles are crucial in assessing fertility. By applying cluster analysis to features extracted from these images (like follicle size, number, and distribution), patients can be categorized into different clusters based on their ovarian reserve or response to stimulation in ART. For instance, one cluster may represent patients with Polycystic Ovary Syndrome (PCOS), characterized by a high number of small follicles, while another cluster might represent patients with a low ovarian reserve.

12.3.2.3 Ovarian Stimulation and Monitoring

- **ML Model:**
  - Ovarian Response Prediction
- **ML Intervention:** During ovarian stimulation, ML models predict the patient's response to drugs before administering drugs, which can help to adjust dosages to optimize egg maturation while minimizing risks of overstimulation.
- **How They Work:**
  - The prediction of ovarian response is a cornerstone of personalized reproductive treatment. By using machine learning models, clinicians can forecast how a patient's ovaries will react to stimulation drugs. This foresight is critical to prevent Ovarian Hyperstimulation Syndrome (OHSS), a serious complication that can occur when the ovaries respond too vigorously.
  - **Example:** The Ovarian Response model could consider a patient's age, hormonal levels, and genetic markers like Single Nucleotide Polymorphisms (SNPs), combined with data from previous treatments, to estimate the ovarian response. This information enables clinicians to adjust the stimulation protocol, accordingly, reducing risks and improving outcomes.

12.3.2.4 Oocyte Retrieval and Sperm Collection

- **ML Models:**
  - Synthetic Data Generation for Image Detection Tasks
  - Sperm Assessment using CASA
  - Oocyte Quality Prediction

- **ML Intervention:** ML assists in assessing the quality of retrieved oocytes and sperm, predicting their viability for successful fertilization.
- **How They Work:**
  - Synthetic Data Generation for Image Detection: Image analysis in ART, especially in sperm, oocyte, and embryo assessment, requires extensive and diverse datasets. However, the availability of such data is often limited due to the rarity of certain conditions and privacy concerns. By using Generative Adversarial Networks (GANs) along with Variational Autoencoders (VAEs), ML can create realistic synthetic images that augment the existing datasets. This approach enhances the training of image recognition models, leading to more accurate and reliable assessments in ART procedures.
  - During the sperm selection process, the CASA system captures real-time images or videos of a sperm sample. The ML model then analyses these visuals, identifying and classifying each sperm cell based on learned patterns. For example, it can distinguish between motile and immotile sperm, and further classify motile as progressive and non-progressive motile, further assess the speed and direction of movement, and evaluate the shape and size of sperm cells. This information is crucial in determining the health and viability of sperm, which directly impacts the success rate of assisted reproductive procedures. Moreover, the system can be trained to adapt to new criteria or improved understanding of sperm health, making it a flexible and evolving tool in the field of reproductive medicine.
  - Recognizing the biomechanical responses of oocytes and embryos to external stimuli during development holds substantial promise, potentially revealing correlations between mechanical responses and developmental potential (Patil et al. 2023; Yanez et al. 2016). The inclusion of quantitative data layers derived from biomechanical characterization could significantly advance ML algorithms and provide a more comprehensive lens for assessing oocyte and embryo quality.

12.3.2.5 In Vitro Fertilization (IVF) Lab Procedures

- **ML Model:**
  - Anomaly Detection with Smart Devices
- **ML Intervention:** ML monitors the IVF lab environment, ensuring optimal conditions for embryo development and alerting staff to any anomalies.
- **How They Work:**
  - In the delicate environment of an IVF lab, even minor fluctuations in temperature, humidity, or equipment performance can impact the success of ART procedures. Smart devices, an ML-driven monitoring system, act as a sentinel for these environments. By continuously analyzing data from various sensors, smart devices can detect and alert staff to any deviations from optimal conditions, allowing for prompt corrective actions.
  - **Example**: Imagine a scenario where smart devices detect a slight but consistent rise in incubator temperature beyond an acceptable threshold. The system

alerts the lab technicians, who then discover a malfunctioning thermostat. Early detection and intervention prevent any adverse effects on the embryos being cultivated.

12.3.2.6 Embryo Culture and Selection

- **ML Models:**
  - Embryo Location Detection
  - Embryo Event Detection
  - Automatic Embryo Grading
- **ML Intervention:** In the critical phase of embryo culture and selection, Machine Learning (ML) algorithms play a transformative role. Utilizing images captured by Time Lapse Monitoring (TLM) Systems, these algorithms are pivotal in analyzing the nuanced development of embryos by detecting embryos in the frame, generating alerts for important events, and selecting the best candidates for transfer based on morphological and developmental criteria.
- **How They Work:**
  - The first model, Embryo Location Detection, begins the process by narrowing down the field of analysis to just the embryos, thus reducing the size of the image for storage and retrieval in further analysis, also making the task more manageable and focused.
  - The Embryo Event Detection model then continuously monitors these identified embryos, using advanced pattern recognition to note significant developmental events. It is adept at recognizing and generating alerts for key developmental milestones in the embryo's growth, such as the transition to different cell stages. This real-time monitoring and alert system ensure that embryologists are informed of critical events in the embryo's development journey. This approach solves the time consuming and inefficient approach of embryologists requiring to manually monitor ~1000 images of an embryo every day to identify significant events.
  - Finally, the Automatic Embryo Grading model applies a set of predefined criteria to grade each embryo, thereby facilitating an informed selection process. This integrated approach not only maximizes the efficiency of the embryologist's work but also significantly improves the accuracy and success rates of the embryo selection process in ART.

12.3.2.7 Embryo Transfer and Implantation

- **ML Models:**
  - Regression
  - Time Series Analysis
- **ML Intervention:** ML models evaluate the readiness of the uterus for implantation, suggesting the best time for embryo transfer.
- **How They Work:**
  - Regression models can assess various factors (endometrial thickness, hormone levels, age, previous ART outcomes) to predict the optimal timing for embryo transfer.

  - Time Series Analysis can be used to track changes in the patient's physiological parameters over time, aiding in determining the best window for implantation.

12.3.2.8 Post-Transfer Monitoring and Pregnancy Test

- **ML Intervention:** After embryo transfer, ML models predict the likelihood of pregnancy, aiding in early detection and management of potential complications.

12.3.2.9 Ongoing Pregnancy Care

- **ML Models:**
  - Longitudinal Data Analysis
  - Predictive Modeling (using Regression Analysis, Survival Analysis)
- **ML Intervention:** Throughout the pregnancy, ML continues to provide insights for personalized care, adjusting treatment plans as needed based on the patient's health data.
- **How They Work:**
  - Longitudinal Data Analysis is used to track and analyze changes in a patient's health parameters throughout the pregnancy.
  - Predictive Modeling, through Regression Analysis, can forecast potential pregnancy complications (like gestational diabetes or preeclampsia) based on ongoing health data. Survival Analysis could be used to estimate the time until specific events or complications might occur, allowing for proactive healthcare management.

12.3.2.10 Delivery and Postpartum Follow-Up

- **ML Intervention:** ML models assist in planning for delivery, including predicting potential risks and preparing for postpartum care.

Case Study: The study (Ramnath Babu et al. 2020) demonstrates the development and application of an ML-based decision-support framework to aid embryologists and clinicians in decision-making during Frozen Embryo Transfer (FET) in In Vitro Fertilization (IVF) treatments, specifically for patients with Polycystic Ovarian Syndrome (PCOS). Traditional approaches in IVF treatments have focused mainly on prediction, without actively aiding in the treatment process. This study shifts the focus to include decision support, using clinical data from 187 PCOS patients who underwent FET-IVF treatment at a single center between 2015 and 2019.

Furthermore, the study highlights the use of the ML Decision Support System. The system can calculate and rank various treatment pathways based on controllable parameters like "Day of freezing", "Culture type", and "Number of embryos transferred", thereby aiding embryologists in choosing the most promising treatment approach.

12.3.3 Conclusion

In every step of a patient's journey in ART, ML intervention offers a tailored, data-driven approach. From initial consultation to successful delivery, these ML models ensure that each decision is backed by comprehensive data analysis, enhancing the chances of a successful outcome. This integrative approach not only improves success rates in ART but also aligns with the vision of personalized medicine, where each patient's unique profile is at the heart of treatment strategies.

12.4 Large Language Models for Reproductive Medicine

The integration of Large Language Models (LLMs) into the realm of reproductive health and medicine represents a significant advancement in the way medical professionals approach diagnosis, treatment, and research in this field. LLMs, with their advanced capabilities in data processing, language understanding, and pattern recognition, offer unprecedented opportunities for enhancing the quality and effectiveness of patient care in ART.

12.4.1 Why LLMs for Reproductive Medicine?

12.4.1.1 Automated Data Analytics for Non-Technical Users

LLMs can democratize access to data analytics in ART, enabling non-technical users like embryologists and clinicians to make data-driven decisions. By inputting raw data into an LLM, users can receive analyses in comprehensible formats.

12.4.1.2 Handling Complex Data

Reproductive medicine generates vast amounts of complex data, including patient medical histories, genomic information, and clinical study results. LLMs are adept at processing and making sense of this data, providing valuable insights that can guide clinical decision-making.

12.4.1.3 Personalized Treatment Approaches

By analyzing patient-specific data, LLMs can aid in developing personalized treatment plans. This is crucial in ART, where individual patient characteristics significantly influence treatment success.

12.4.1.4 Research and Development

LLMs can rapidly review and synthesize existing medical literature, aiding in research and keeping practitioners up to date with the latest advancements in reproductive medicine.

12.4.1.5 Enhancing Patient Engagement

LLMs can be used to create more engaging and informative patient interactions, helping individuals understand their treatment options and what to expect throughout their ART journey.

12.4.1.6 Scenario

An embryologist inputs ovarian stimulation response data into the LLM system, which then analyzes the data against a vast repository of similar cases and provides insights on the likely outcomes and recommendations for future protocols.

12.4.2 What Is an LLM?

Large Language Models (LLMs) are advanced artificial intelligence systems that have been trained to understand, generate, and interact with human language. These models are based on deep learning techniques, specifically neural networks, which enable them to process and analyze vast amounts of text data.

- **Scale and Capability:** LLMs are "large" both in terms of the size of the neural networks (often consisting of billions of parameters) and the extensive datasets they are trained on. This scale allows them to have a broad understanding of language and context.
- **Applications:** LLMs are used in a variety of applications, including natural language processing tasks like translation, summarization, question-answering, and conversational agents.

12.4.3 Pre-Trained Foundational Models

A foundational model refers to a large-scale, pre-trained model that serves as a base upon which further specialized models can be built. These models are foundational in the sense that they provide a broad and versatile understanding of language, patterns, or data, which can then be adapted or fine-tuned for more specific tasks or domains.

12.4.4 Pre-Trained Foundational Models vs. Fine-Tuning

- **Pre-Trained Models:** These are models that have been previously trained on large, diverse datasets. This training enables the model to understand and generate human language. However, pre-trained models are often generalists, having broad knowledge but not specialized in any domain.
- **Fine-Tuning:** This process involves additional training of a pre-trained model on a specific dataset. Fine-tuning tailors the model to be more adept at handling language and tasks specific to a particular domain or application.

12.4.5 Process of Fine-Tuning LLMs for ART

12.4.5.1 The Importance of Reinforcement Learning from Human Feedback (RLHF)

Reinforcement Learning from Human Feedback (RLHF) is a critical component in the fine-tuning process of LLMs, especially when adapting these models to specialized fields such as reproductive medicine. RLHF serves several key purposes:

- **Improving Model Accuracy and Relevance:** Through RLHF, human experts provide feedback on the model's outputs, guiding the model to generate more accurate and contextually relevant responses.
- **Addressing Complex and Nuanced Queries:** In reproductive medicine, queries often involve complex medical terminology and require nuanced understanding. RLHF helps in training the model to better understand and respond to such specialized queries.
- **Mitigating Biases and Errors:** Human feedback is essential in identifying and correcting biases or errors that might be present in the model's initial training data. This ensures that the model's advice or insights are balanced and unbiased.
- **Ensuring Ethical and Responsible AI Use:** Involving medical professionals in the RLHF process ensures that the model adheres to ethical standards and aligns with clinical best practices, making it a responsible AI tool for healthcare.

12.4.5.2 Fine-Tuning LLMs for Reproductive Medicine with RLHF

Selecting a Suitable Base Model

- Choose a robust pre-trained LLM that best aligns with the needs of reproductive medicine in terms of language capabilities and initial training data.

Curating a Specialized Dataset

- Collect and prepare a dataset specifically tailored to reproductive medicine, including clinical studies, patient records, treatment protocols, and recent research findings.

Data Preprocessing and Annotation

- Clean, preprocess, and, if necessary, annotate the dataset to ensure high-quality, relevant input for the fine-tuning process.

Initial Fine-Tuning Process

- Utilize the prepared dataset to start the fine-tuning process, adjusting the model to better understand and respond to domain-specific queries and information.

Incorporating Prompt Engineering

- **Prompt Development:** Concurrently with or immediately following the initial fine-tuning, develop a set of targeted prompts that reflect typical queries and tasks relevant to reproductive medicine.

- **Testing and Refinement:** Test these prompts with the fine-tuned model, refining them based on the model's responses to ensure they effectively guide the model towards providing accurate and relevant information.
- **Diverse Scenario Coverage:** Ensure the prompts cover a wide range of topics within reproductive medicine to prepare the model for various real-world applications.

Implementing RLHF

- **Feedback Loop:** Engage reproductive medicine experts to review and provide feedback on the model's outputs. This feedback should focus on the accuracy, relevance, and medical appropriateness of the responses.
- **Iterative Learning:** Incorporate this expert feedback into the model's training regimen, allowing it to learn from its mistakes and improve its understanding of the domain.
- **Validation and Adjustment:** Regularly validate the model's performance with real-world scenarios and adjust the training based on expert feedback.

12.4.6 The Importance of User Interface in Popularizing LLMs

The interface of an LLM plays a crucial role in its adoption and usability. Early LLMs, while powerful, were often relegated to research and development due to their complex interfaces. The advent of user-friendly interfaces, as seen in ChatGPT, has changed this landscape dramatically.

Example: ChatGPT's conversational interface made it accessible to a broad audience, including medical professionals who may not have technical expertise in AI. In ART, such an interface allows for easy querying of patient data, interpretation of medical literature, and even assists in drafting patient communication, making the technology a valuable asset in everyday clinical practice.

12.4.7 Conclusion

The incorporation of Large Language Models (LLMs) into ART goes beyond mere data analysis; it opens up new avenues for interaction and knowledge acquisition for both clinicians and patients. For clinicians, LLMs serve as a powerful tool for interpreting complex medical data, staying updated with the latest research, and making informed decisions about patient care. Patients, on the other hand, stand to benefit significantly from this technology. LLMs can offer personalized responses to patient queries, provide explanations about treatment options in understandable language, and assist in navigating the often-complex journey of reproductive treatments. This not only enhances patient knowledge and understanding of their treatment but also fosters a greater sense of involvement and empowerment in their healthcare journey.

Furthermore, the interactive nature of LLMs, enhanced by fine-tuning and prompt engineering, ensures that the information provided is tailored to the specific context of each patient and clinician interaction. The future of ART, augmented with the capabilities of LLMs, looks towards a more informed, interactive, and patient-centric approach to fertility care.

12.5 Federated Learning in Reproductive Health and Medicine

12.5.1 Why Federated Learning in ART?

12.5.1.1 A Paradigm Shift in Data Handling and Analysis

Federated Learning represents a transformative approach in the realm of ART. At its core, Federated Learning upholds the principle that ***Data does not leave the Clinic***, a crucial factor in a field where confidentiality is paramount. This novel method of data handling and analysis addresses significant privacy concerns and sets the stage for a new era of collaborative learning.

12.5.1.2 Privacy and Confidentiality

In ART, patient data is not just sensitive; it's often the most critical factor in treatment decisions. Federated Learning ensures that this data remains within the clinic, mitigating risks associated with data breaches and unauthorized access. This level of privacy fosters patient trust and compliance, essential elements in reproductive healthcare.

12.5.1.3 Collaborative Learning from Diverse Datasets

Federated Learning's true strength lies in its ability to facilitate learning from a vast array of datasets without compromising individual clinic's data sovereignty. Clinics with different specializations and patient demographics can contribute to a broader understanding of reproductive health issues.

Example: Clinic A's in-depth experience in dealing with Polycystic Ovary Syndrome (PCOS) and Clinic B's expertise in male infertility can complement each other through Federated Learning. Both clinics benefit from shared insights, leading to more comprehensive care for a broader range of conditions.

12.5.1.4 Decentralized Data Analysis for Robust Insights

Unlike traditional models where data is centralized, Federated Learning leverages decentralized data. This approach allows for the aggregation of diverse insights, enhancing the understanding of complex ART treatments and patient responses. Such a decentralized model is particularly advantageous in ART, where individual patient responses can vary significantly.

12.5.1.5 Enhanced Patient Outcomes Through Collaborative Efforts

With Federated Learning, clinics can pool their insights to develop better ML Decision Support Systems, more effective treatment protocols, and personalized patient care strategies. This collaboration can lead to higher success rates in treatments and a deeper understanding of factors affecting fertility.

Case Study: The study (Sheller et al. 2020) explores the efficacy of Federated Learning in Medicine. The study shows that federated learning emerges as a promising approach for data-private, multi-institutional collaborations, allowing for model training across various institutions without the need to share patient data directly. The study suggests that adopting federated learning in clinical settings could lead to the development of models trained on significantly larger datasets, thereby enhancing precision and personalized medicine.

12.5.2 What Is Federated Learning?

Federated Learning is a machine learning approach that enables multiple collaborators, such as multiple hospitals or research centers, to collaboratively contribute towards developing shared ML models without exchanging the actual data. Essentially, instead of sending data to a central location, Federated Learning brings the algorithm to the data. This method ensures that sensitive information remains at its source, addressing privacy and security concerns.

12.5.2.1 The Mechanics of Federated Learning

In Federated Learning, a shared ML model is sent to each participant (e.g., clinics or research labs). Each participant trains the model on their local data and then sends only the model updates (not the data itself) back to a central server. The server aggregates these updates to improve the shared model, which is then redistributed to all participants. This cycle continues until the model is optimally trained. Figure 12.2 provides an overview diagram of Federated Learning in IVF clinics, illustrating how this collaborative approach enables the development of robust ML models while preserving data privacy.

12.5.3 Analogy with UPI's Consent Layer

12.5.3.1 Comparative Analysis with UPI

The one-time consent model in Unified Payments Interface (UPI) transactions provides a useful analogy for understanding Federated Learning in ART. In UPI systems, users give their consent once for their financial data to be used for transactions, simplifying, and securing the process. Similarly, a one-time consent model for medical data usage in ART can streamline data collection, reduce bureaucratic hurdles, and enhance patient participation.

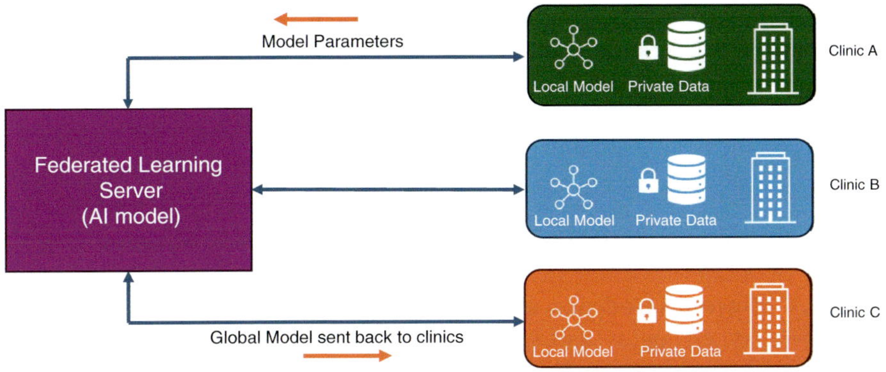

Fig. 12.2 Overview diagram of federated learning in IVF clinics, illustrating how this collaborative approach enables the development of robust ML models while preserving data privacy

12.5.3.2 Benefits of a One-Time Consent Model

This model can significantly improve the efficiency and scope of medical research and treatment. With patients' consent, their anonymized data can contribute to a larger dataset, enabling more robust research and improved outcomes in ART.

12.5.4 Enhanced Patient Services Through a Central Data Repository

12.5.4.1 Structure and Management

The central data repository in a Federated Learning system acts as the brain of the operation. Though it doesn't store patient data directly, it aggregates insights derived from various clinics' analyses. This Insights Hub must be meticulously managed to ensure data integrity, security, and compliance with regulatory standards.

12.5.4.2 Rapid Learning and Identification of Outliers

The repository facilitates rapid learning across different clinical environments. By pooling insights, it can identify common patterns and outliers more effectively than any single clinic could. This can lead to breakthroughs in understanding infertility causes and treatment responses.

12.5.4.3 Tailoring Treatments with Data-Driven Insights

One of the most significant benefits of a central data repository in Federated Learning is the ability to tailor treatments based on comprehensive data-driven insights. By analyzing vast amounts of anonymized data from various clinics, practitioners can identify the most effective treatment protocols for specific conditions, leading to higher success rates in ART.

12.5.4.4 Improving Access and Quality of Care

The central repository can also enhance the overall quality and accessibility of reproductive healthcare. For instance, clinics in remote or under-resourced areas can access insights derived from larger, more diverse datasets, leveling the playing field and providing high-quality care regardless of location.

12.5.5 Empowering Patients Through Data Contribution

12.5.5.1 Informed Decision Making

In a Federated Learning system, patients are not just passive data providers; they are active participants in a larger healthcare ecosystem. By contributing their data, they empower not just themselves but also others by enhancing the collective understanding of reproductive health.

12.5.5.2 The Ripple Effect of Shared Knowledge

As patients contribute their anonymized data, they benefit from the collective knowledge gained from others' experiences. This shared knowledge pool can lead to more informed choices and personalized treatment plans, effectively creating a virtuous cycle of learning and improvement.

12.5.6 Challenges, Considerations, and Future Perspectives

12.5.6.1 Navigating Data Privacy Concerns

Despite the benefits, Federated Learning in ART faces significant challenges, chiefly regarding data privacy. Ensuring that patient data remains secure and anonymized requires robust protocols and continuous vigilance. Addressing these concerns is paramount to maintaining trust and efficacy in the system.

12.5.6.2 Collaborative Efforts Across Borders

To maximize the potential of Federated Learning in ART, collaboration across clinics, countries, and disciplines is necessary. Sharing knowledge and best practices can help overcome regional disparities in reproductive healthcare and foster global improvements.

12.5.6.3 Integrating Future Perspectives

Looking ahead, the integration of advanced analytics, AI, and machine learning in Federated Learning systems holds immense promise. These technologies could further refine data analysis, leading to even more personalized and effective ART treatments. Moreover, as regulatory bodies and governments understand the potential of FL, we can anticipate more supportive policies and frameworks that encourage innovation while safeguarding patient interests.

12.5.7 Conclusion

Federated Learning in ART is at a pivotal juncture, poised to revolutionize reproductive healthcare. By addressing its challenges head-on and embracing its potential, we can look forward to a future where data-driven insights lead to more successful, personalized, and patient-centric reproductive treatments.

12.6 Genome Sequence Modelling in Reproductive Health and Medicine

The advent of genome sequence modelling can revolutionize our understanding and approach to fertility, genetic disorders, and prenatal care. This section delves into the transformative potential of this technology, shedding light on its applications and future implications.

12.6.1 Integration of Genomic Data and Machine Learning

The integration of vast genomic datasets with advanced machine learning algorithms has opened new avenues in reproductive medicine. For example, researchers at the Broad Institute (Williams 2023) have leveraged machine learning to predict the likelihood of genetic disorders, using data derived from thousands of genome sequences. This predictive capability is invaluable in assessing the risk of inheritable conditions, enabling more informed reproductive decisions.

12.6.2 Embryo Selection and Genetic Screening

In Vitro Fertilization (IVF) procedures are increasingly incorporating genome sequence modelling for embryo selection. Techniques such as Preimplantation Genetic Diagnosis (PGD) and Preimplantation Genetic Screening (PGS) are being enhanced by machine learning algorithms, which can analyze genetic data from embryos to identify those with the highest potential for a successful pregnancy and the lowest risk of genetic abnormalities.

12.6.3 Genome Sequence LLMs in Reproductive Health

LLMs in genomics function by transforming genetic data into a format akin to natural language, allowing for more intuitive analysis and predictions. For instance, Hyena DNA (Nguyen et al. 2023), DNABert (Ji et al. 2021), and DNABert-2 (Zhou et al. 2023) are genome foundational models which can act as the base models.

Fine-tuning them using ART datasets allows for the creation of highly specialized tools tailored to address specific challenges in reproductive medicine. By integrating these fine-tuned models into clinical settings, practitioners can gain unprecedented insights into genetic factors influencing fertility, embryo development, and potential genetic disorders, leading to more effective and personalized reproductive healthcare strategies.

12.6.4 Conclusion

While the benefits are substantial, genome sequence modelling in reproductive health also raises ethical concerns. The prospect of "designer babies", where genetic selection may extend beyond health considerations to physical or cognitive traits, poses significant ethical dilemmas. Collaborative efforts between geneticists, data scientists, and clinicians are crucial in translating these technological advancements into meaningful healthcare solutions.

12.7 Research to Production

12.7.1 Adoption of Technologies in Reproductive Medicine

The adoption of advanced technologies in reproductive medicine has been transformative. However, the journey from research to clinical implementation is complex, influenced by factors like technological readiness, regulatory compliance, and clinical validation. Let's delve into specific technologies:

- **Blockchain in Data Hub:** Implementing blockchain for secure data management in healthcare is a gradual process, often slowed by technological complexity and the need for substantial infrastructural changes.
- **ML Decision Support Systems:** These systems' adoption hinges on demonstrating clinical efficacy and ensuring integration with existing healthcare infrastructures.
- **Large Language Models (LLM):** LLMs face adoption challenges related to interpretability and ethical use of AI. The time frame for adoption is longer, given the need for rigorous validation of their clinical relevance.
- **Federated Learning:** This approach's adoption is relatively quicker as it addresses crucial data privacy concerns, a significant barrier in healthcare technology.
- **Genome Sequence Modelling:** These models have a longer developmental timeline due to the intricate nature of genomic data and the necessity for extensive testing to ensure accuracy and ethical considerations in genetic testing.

12.7.2 MLOps and LLMOps in Reproductive Medicine: Lifecycle and Best Practices

MLOps (Machine Learning Operations) is the foundational framework that ensures the smooth functioning of widely used services like Google Maps, Amazon's recommendation system, Instagram's news feed, and Netflix's viewing suggestions. It encompasses the comprehensive management of machine learning models from creation to deployment and ongoing maintenance. For instance, in Google Maps, MLOps is responsible for the constant updating and scaling of algorithms to provide real-time navigation. MLOps involves managing and automating the lifecycle of machine learning models. It ensures these models are efficiently developed, deployed, and maintained.

LLMOps (Large Language Model Operations) plays a crucial role in making tools like ChatGPT accessible and efficient for end-users. LLMOps manages the lifecycle of large language models, which includes the development, deployment, updating, and monitoring of these models to ensure they function effectively. For ChatGPT, LLMOps ensures that the model not only generates accurate and contextually appropriate responses but also does so consistently for a vast number of users at any given time. This involves optimizing the model's performance to handle diverse queries and interactions while maintaining ethical and responsible usage standards.

12.7.2.1 Combined Lifecycle of ML and LLM Projects

The lifecycle of both Machine Learning (ML) and Large Language Models (LLMs) in reproductive medicine (Fig. 12.3) follows a similar trajectory with distinct nuances.

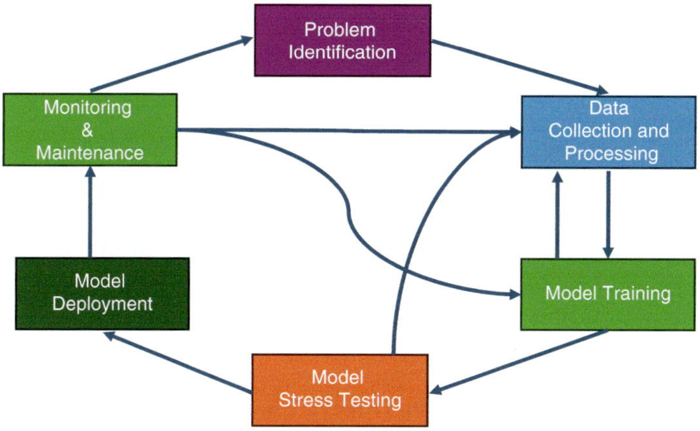

Fig. 12.3 The lifecycle of both machine learning (ML) and large language models (LLMs) in reproductive medicine

The lifecycle typically includes the following:

- **Problem Identification:** Determining specific challenges or opportunities in reproductive medicine where ML or LLM can be applied.
- **Data Acquisition and Preparation:** Collecting and preparing relevant data, which is particularly sensitive in reproductive health, ensuring privacy and ethical considerations.
- **Model Training**: Building and training the model. For LLMs, this involves handling larger datasets and more complex architectures. Interpretation at this stage helps in identifying if the model is making predictions for the right reasons, which is particularly important in healthcare applications.
- **Model Validation and Testing:** Rigorously testing the model for accuracy, reliability, and ethical compliance, which is crucial in the healthcare domain. During this stage, the model's behavior will prompt several iterations back to the Data Acquisition and Preparation phase.
- **Model Deployment:** Integrating the model into the clinical workflow. This phase requires careful planning to ensure minimal disruption and maximum utility.
- **Data & Model Monitoring and Maintenance:** Continuously monitoring the data drift and model's performance in real-world scenarios and updating it as necessary. This stage will involve looping back to either the Data Collection or the Model Training phase, depending on the requirements identified during the process.

12.7.2.2 Best Practices in Operations

When it comes to operations, the practices for ML and LLMs converge and diverge based on the project's needs:

- **Continuous Integration and Continuous Deployment (CI/CD):** Regularly updating models with new data and algorithms is crucial. For LLMs, this might involve more frequent updates due to their complexity and evolving capabilities.
- **Scalability and Resource Management:** Efficiently managing resources is critical, especially for LLMs, which require more computational power.
- **Security and Compliance:** Ensuring data security and compliance with healthcare regulations. For LLMs, this also involves managing the risks associated with the generation of sensitive information.
- **Ethical AI Practices:** Upholding ethical standards in AI applications, with a particular focus on transparency and fairness.

12.7.2.3 The Importance of a Feedback Loop

A robust feedback loop is vital in both MLOps and LLMOps for several reasons:

- **Continuous Improvement:** Feedback from real-world applications helps in fine-tuning models, making them more accurate and reliable over time.

- **Adaptability:** In the dynamic field of reproductive medicine, where new research and findings are common, feedback loops help models adapt to new knowledge and changing practices.
- **Patient-Centric Approach:** Patient outcomes and experiences provide invaluable insights, enabling models to become more patient-focused and effective in clinical settings.
- **Collaboration Enhancement:** Feedback loops encourage collaboration between clinicians, data scientists, and patients, fostering a holistic approach to healthcare solutions.

While LLMs and ML offer transformative potential in data analysis, patient interaction, and medical research, they come with substantial resource requirements.

12.7.2.4 Factors Contributing to High Operating Costs in ML and LLMs

- **Computational Resources:** Both LLMs and MLOps demand significant computational power. LLMs require it for training and inference processes, especially when handling large medical datasets. MLOps, encompassing the entire lifecycle of machine learning models, also requires robust hardware for model development, testing, and deployment.
- **Energy Consumption:** The energy demands for running LLMs are notably high due to their iterative training over extensive datasets. Similarly, the continuous integration and deployment processes in MLOps contribute to increased energy usage.
- **Data Storage and Management:** Storing and managing the vast volumes of data essential for LLMs and MLOps add to operational costs. This includes expenses related to secure and compliant data storage solutions, especially crucial in handling sensitive medical data.
- **Maintenance and Updates:** Regular updating and maintenance of both LLMs and machine learning models under MLOps are essential for their accuracy and relevance. This ongoing investment includes costs for skilled personnel such as data scientists and ML engineers.
- **Scalability Costs:** As the application of these technologies expands in healthcare, scaling them to meet growing data and operational demands further increases expenses.

12.7.2.5 Implications in Reproductive Medicine

In reproductive medicine, LLMs and MLOps present opportunities for enhancing patient care and advancing medical research. However, the high operational costs necessitate a careful evaluation of their value proposition. These technologies must demonstrate tangible benefits, such as improved patient outcomes and efficiencies in medical processes, to justify the investment.

Healthcare providers and research institutions need to balance the advanced capabilities of LLMs and MLOps with the economic aspects of healthcare delivery. Efficient model architectures, cloud-based solutions, and collaborative funding and resource-sharing models can be effective strategies to manage costs while leveraging the advantages of these cutting-edge technologies in reproductive medicine.

12.7.3 Conclusion

Transitioning from research to production in reproductive medicine, particularly through data-driven technologies, requires a nuanced understanding of each technology's development timeline, cost-benefit profile, and operational best practices. MLOps and LLMOps play a pivotal role in ensuring these technologies are effectively integrated into clinical settings, driving forward the future of reproductive health.

12.8 Chapter Conclusion

Central themes include the strategic shift towards personalized, data-driven approaches in assisted reproduction, and the integration of predictive modeling, data synthesis, genomic insights, and language processing, all underpinned by stringent data security measures. These advancements herald a new paradigm of patient-centric, ethically sound practices, poised to redefine care standards and success in assisted reproduction. The chapter encapsulates the holistic vision of future reproductive medicine, emphasizing the collective ushering of this new era.

Acknowledgments The authors would like to acknowledge the use of AI-based tools such as Quillbot and Grammarly to improve readability and summarize some parts of the text. The authors have further reviewed the text and take full responsibility for the text.

Conflict of Interest The authors have no conflicts of interest to declare that are relevant to the content of this chapter.

References

Buterin V (2015) [PDF] A next generation smart contract & decentralized application platform | Semantic Scholar. https://www.semanticscholar.org/paper/A-NEXT-GENERATION-SMART-CONTRACT-%26-DECENTRALIZED-Buterin/0dbb8a54ca5066b82fa086bbf5db4c54b947719a. Accessed 27 Mar 2024

Data Hub - Family Planning 2030. https://www.fp2030.org/data-hub/. Accessed 27 Mar 2024

Davis N (2024) UK fertility treatment comparison tool featuring IVF data launched. The Guardian

Gliklich RE, Leavy MB, Dreyer NA (2020) Registries for evaluating patient outcomes: a user's guide. Agency for Healthcare Research and Quality (AHRQ)

Gordon WJ, Catalini C (2018) Blockchain technology for healthcare: facilitating the transition to patient-driven interoperability. Comput Struct Biotechnol J 16:224–230. https://doi.org/10.1016/j.csbj.2018.06.003

Iansiti M, Lakhani KR (2017) The truth about Blockchain. Harvard Business Review

Ji Y, Zhou Z, Liu H, Davuluri RV (2021) DNABERT: pre-trained bidirectional encoder representations from transformers model for DNA-language in genome. Bioinformatics 37:2112–2120. https://doi.org/10.1093/bioinformatics/btab083

Kuo T-T, Kim H-E, Ohno-Machado L (2017) Blockchain distributed ledger technologies for biomedical and health care applications. J Am Med Inform Assoc 24:1211–1220. https://doi.org/10.1093/jamia/ocx068

Mettler M (2016) Blockchain technology in healthcare: the revolution starts here. In: 2016 IEEE 18th international conference on e-health networking, applications and services (Healthcom). IEEE, Munich, pp 1–3

Ministry of Law and Justice (Legislative Department) (2023) The Digital PERSONAL Data Protection Act. https://www.meity.gov.in/writereaddata/files/Digital%20Personal%20Data%20Protection%20Act%202023.pdf

Nakamoto S (2008) Bitcoin: a peer-to-peer electronic cash system. https://bitcoin.org/bitcoin.pdf

Nguyen E, Poli M, Faizi M et al (2023) HyenaDNA: long-range genomic sequence modeling at single nucleotide resolution. https://doi.org/10.48550/ARXIV.2306.15794

NIMH Data Archive - ABCD. https://nda.nih.gov/abcd. Accessed 27 Mar 2024

Patil KD, Kumar P, Bharadwaj KKS et al (2023) Bulk stiffness and recovery time—a measure of development of mouse embryos. JRHM 4:4. https://doi.org/10.25259/JRHM_26_2022

Ramnath Babu TJ, Roy VS, Jambunath Y et al (2020) A machine-learning (ML) based decision support framework with a case study in frozen-embryo-transfer (FET) in-vitro-fertilization (IVF) for patients with polycystic ovarian syndrome (PCOS). In: ESHRE 2020—abstract book. European Society of Human Reproduction and Embryology

Rana G (2024) Research guides: global sexual and reproductive health: data sources. https://guides.lib.umich.edu/global_srh/data. Accessed 27 Mar 2024

Sheller MJ, Edwards B, Reina GA et al (2020) Federated learning in medicine: facilitating multi-institutional collaborations without sharing patient data. Sci Rep 10:12598. https://doi.org/10.1038/s41598-020-69250-1

Tapscott D, Tapscott A (2016) Blockchain revolution: how the technology behind bitcoin is changing money, business, and the world. Penguin Publishing Group

Williams SCP (2023) Artificial intelligence system predicts consequences of disruptions to genetic networks. In: Broad Institute. https://www.broadinstitute.org/news/artificial-intelligence-system-predicts-consequences-disruptions-genetic-networks. Accessed 27 Mar 2024

Yanez LZ, Han J, Behr BB et al (2016) Human oocyte developmental potential is predicted by mechanical properties within hours after fertilization. Nat Commun 7:10809. https://doi.org/10.1038/ncomms10809

Zhou Z, Ji Y, Li W et al (2023) DNABERT-2: efficient foundation model and benchmark for multi-species genome. https://doi.org/10.48550/ARXIV.2306.15006

Printed by Printforce, the Netherl